The plan that will change your life

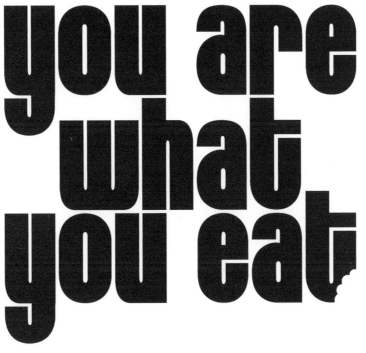

Dr. Gillian McKeith

Based on the Celador Production of *You Are What You Eat*

DUTTON

This book is dedicated to my two wee lassies.
Hugs, love and kisses from Mummy. Eat your greens!!

DUTTON
Published by Penguin Group (USA) Inc.
375 Hudson Street, New York, New York 10014, U.S.A.
Penguin Group (Canada), 10 Alcorn Avenue, Toronto, Ontario, Canada M4V 3B2 (a division of Pearson Penguin Canada Inc.); Penguin Books Ltd, 80 Strand, London WC2R 0RL, England; Penguin Ireland, 25 St Stephen's Green, Dublin 2, Ireland (a division of Penguin Books Ltd); Penguin Group (Australia), 250 Camberwell Road, Camberwell, Victoria 3124, Australia (a division of Pearson Australia Group Pty Ltd); Penguin Books India Pvt Ltd, 11 Community Centre, Panchsheel Park, New Dehli - 110 017, India; Penguin Group (NZ), cnr Airborne and Rosedale Roads, Albany, Auckland 1310, New Zealand (a division of Pearson New Zealand Ltd); Penguin Books (South Africa) (Pty) Ltd, 24 Sturdee Avenue, Rosebank, Johannesburg 2196, South Africa

Penguin Books Ltd, Registered Offices: 80 Strand, London WC2R 0RL, England

Published by Dutton, a member of Penguin Group (USA) Inc.
Originally published in the UK by Michael Joseph, an imprint of the Penguin Group.

First American printing, April 2005
10 9 8 7 6 5 4 3 2 1

LIBRARY OF CONGRESS CATALOGING-IN-PUBLICATION DATA
has been applied for.

ISBN 0-525-94891-0

Printed in the United States of America
Designed by Smith & Gilmour, London

CONTENTS

MY STORY

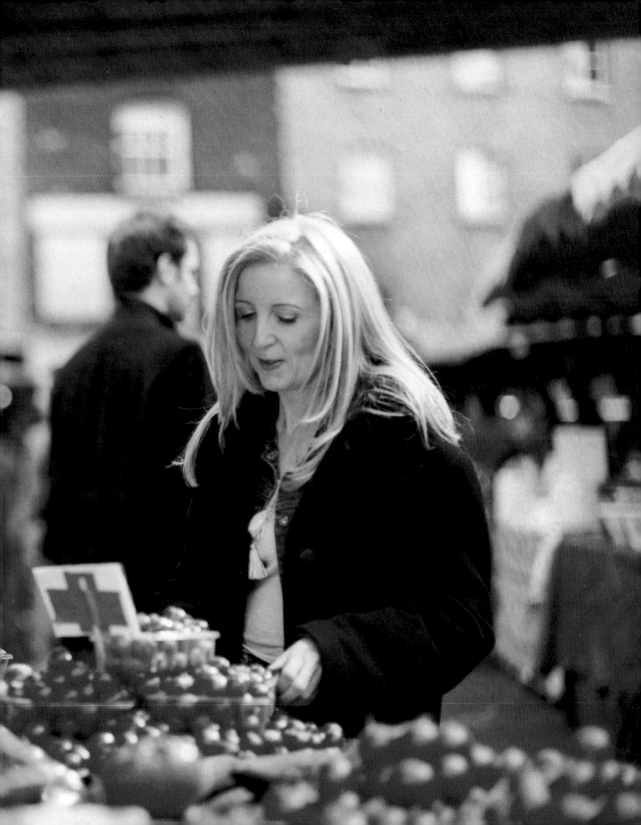

Some people paint me as the unrepentant ruthless nutritionist, obsessed with natural foods and healthy diet. My own mother is afraid to spend Christmas dinner with me, because she is worried that I'll start lecturing her on good food and bad food, and my daughter has been known to call me a "food freak."

Okay, I admit it. I am passionate about what goes into your body. I wasn't always like this though. Years ago I ate only foods that were frozen, or in a plastic package, and I could not get through the day without my daily ration of chips and chocolate bars. Growing up in the Highlands of Scotland, I loved my diet of mince and potatoes, fish and chips, custard and jam rolls.

And then I fell in love with an American, a health nut. I went to live near his home in Philadelphia, but I refused to let his weird ways influence my normal lifestyle. That is, until my twenty-fourth birthday, which is when everything changed. My boyfriend surprised me with an envelope. All it said on the card was that I was "going on a long journey to a special place" on my special day. At that very moment, I had no idea as to just how long my journey would be. We jumped in the car and began the very long drive to an undisclosed location. During the six-hour-long drive, I imagined luxury hotel rooms with hot tubs, perhaps overlooking the mountains or prairie, by a river or a hot spring. After a few hours on the highway, I spotted a sign blaring, "New York State Welcomes You." I then started to imagine visiting the Empire State Building, Broadway, the Statue of Liberty, staying on Fifth Avenue or Madison Avenue. My heart was pounding with anticipation. This Scottish lassie was on her way to the "Big Apple" in this big country with this big man. Wow, what a birthday!

Just before the seventh hour we arrived at our destination. No Big Apple, no mountains and certainly no hot tub in sight.

"We are going to a macrobiotic lunch for your birthday," Mr. America shockingly gushes.

"To a what?" I shoot back.

"You'll see," he calmly assures.

We entered a ramshackle hut filled with dozens of people sitting around makeshift folding tables and folding chairs with paper plates and plastic forks. The setting looked more appropriate for a children's tea party, but here were adults of all ages, clearly from all walks of life; some dressed smartly and sophisticated, others casual and relaxed. Was my boyfriend part of some scary cult? I wondered. My parents warned me about things like this before I left Scotland.

The program finally commences. The keynote speaker, Elaine Nussbaum, a slight, soft-spoken slender lady with the most sincere eyes and a strong New York accent and author of a small underground book, titled *Recovery*, is introduced. She begins to tell her story and it turns out to be the most profound story of my life. I listen in disbelief first, then awe, and finally inspiration and hope.

Elaine was given two weeks to live. Every bone in her body had been riddled with cancer and she could barely walk, talk, breathe, sit or stand. The hospital sent her home to die. They could do no more for her.

On her deathbed, a friend decided to spoon-feed her an esoteric diet, called "macrobiotic." This incorporated natural vegetarian foods like brown rice, green vegetables, seeds, seaweeds, beans and lots of soy or "miso" soups. Within one month, Elaine began to regain strength. Within two months, she felt like she was no longer ill.

She then went back to the hospital for tests and the doctors discovered that her cancer had disappeared in full. They had never seen anything like it, and I had never heard of anything so incredible.

That's when my journey began, when I realized just how powerful food is. We indeed are what we eat. I was suffering with a litany of normal health complaints that we all know too well when we work and play too hard. I had headaches, tiredness, body pains, aches, pimples on my face. I suffered from candidiasis, an insidious yeast infection, and I was over my ideal body weight. When I stopped long enough to genuinely think about it, I realized that I was one of the least healthy persons I knew.

Today I see the same parallels with my own patients at the McKeith Clinic in London. When patients first arrive, they are usually poor eaters, many are overweight, and some are at crisis point. My goal with you, as with my patients, is to get you to know what is best for you to eat, and which foods will help you to lose weight, stay slim and improve your health for life.

You really can do it if you follow my plan. Do much of what I tell you most of the time, and you will surely be healthier, fitter, stronger, sexier and happier. That's my promise to you. I have treated literally thousands of people with fantastic, unprecedented results. People will travel from every region of the globe to get help. I've seen patients from just about every nationality and walk of life, including Hollywood stars, royalty, world leaders, soccer players and Olympic athletes. But they're mostly people like you and me. And they all have one thing in common: All of them, regardless of their background, are made up of what they eat! And those who eat horribly are generally, and not surprisingly, sicker than those who eat healthily.

My patients often have different goals: the athlete, for example, may want to achieve better performance; the housewife may need more energy; the office worker may need to strengthen adrenal glands to be able to handle stress; the elderly man may need more constitutional support, and so on. But in every case, the food that goes in becomes the body's medicine, and if you feed your body the wrong stuff it'll simply lay down fat, lower your energy, sex drive, even your brain power.

In picking up this book you have taken the all-important first step on the road back to a slimmer, healthier you. You can choose the wrong drug or my correct prescription. It's your choice, but if you make the right decision your body is really going to thank you for it. And this is a prescription for the whole family too, so don't feel isolated. It's simply going to be about changing a few habits and recognizing the harm that certain foods are inflicting on you.

After more than fifteen years in clinical practice, I have found that the people who take decent care of their bodies, and eat the right foods, are generally the healthiest specimens. They are stabilized at their natural, healthy weight, plus they are more energized, have better sex lives, are more relaxed about life, enjoy smarter brain function and are even, on balance, happier. This can be you too.

To a large extent, this book is about discovery and knowledge. If I can educate you and turn you on to the right foods, then you will have the best chance of being slim, well and healthy. I want you to benefit from my many years of research and successful treatments on thousands of people. Anyone can do it – just let me show you how.

Gillian M. Keith

Dr. Gillian McKeith
April 2005

CHAPTER 1

YOU ARE WHAT YOU EAT

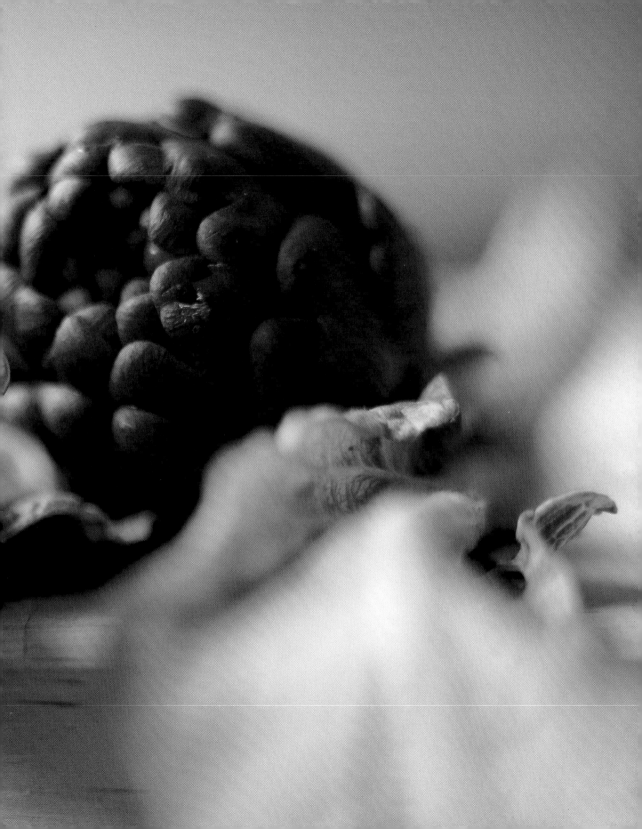

THE FOOD WE EAT IS LIKE FUEL. IT GIVES OUR BODIES THE ENERGY THEY NEED TO FUNCTION WELL. IF YOU DON'T MAKE SURE THAT THE FUEL YOU PUMP INTO YOUR BODY IS OF THE RIGHT QUALITY OR QUANTITY, YOU JUST WON'T FEEL AS HEALTHY AS YOU COULD.

WE ALL HAVE UP TO 100 TRILLION CELLS IN OUR BODIES, EACH ONE DEMANDING A CONSTANT SUPPLY OF DAILY NUTRIENTS IN ORDER TO FUNCTION OPTIMALLY. FOOD AFFECTS ALL THOSE CELLS, AND BY EXTENSION EVERY ASPECT OF OUR BEING: MOOD, ENERGY LEVELS, FOOD CRAVINGS, THINKING CAPACITY, SEX DRIVE, SLEEPING HABITS AND GENERAL HEALTH. IN SHORT, HEALTHY EATING IS THE KEY TO WELL-BEING.

THE EVIDENCE

The first step to turning around your life and your health was in picking up this book. But how can I now convince you to take the all-important next steps and break your bad diet habits?

The relationship between food and health is significant. Diet plays a vital part in promoting good health and well-being. The first crucial step is to make the connection between good food choices and good health, and poor food choices and bad health.

I realized this when I looked at the food diaries of the participants for my TV show, *You Are What You Eat*. Not only were all participants overweight at the beginning of the series but they all had other health complaints, many of which were caused by the poor food choices they made. These foods were the catalyst for most ailments and complaints. When I prepared a table of the bad foods that they had eaten for a week and explained how these foods affected the body, the relationship between food and health suddenly became shockingly apparent.

HERE ARE TEN IMPORTANT FOOD FACTS:

1 A diet high in fat (particularly saturated fat) and high in salt is associated with an increased risk of coronary heart disease.

2 It is estimated that, on average, a third of cancers could be prevented by changes in diet. A diet which is high in fiber and whole grain cereal and low in fat has the potential to prevent a number of cancers, including colon, stomach and breast cancer.

3 Many fertility experts believe that an unhealthy diet, high in fat, sugar, and processed foods and low in nutrients essential to fertility, can lead to infertility and increase the chances of miscarriage.

4 A diet high in fat, sugar and salt leads to weight gain and increases the risk of obesity. Carrying excess weight doesn't just increase the risk of heart disease, diabetes, cancer and infertility, it is also associated with fatigue, low self-esteem and poor mental and physical performance.

5 An unhealthy diet increases the risk of depression and mood swings. It's also linked to PMS, food cravings and anxiety.

6 A diet high in additives, preservatives and refined sugar can cause poor concentration, hyperactivity and aggression. This is because foods high in sugar and additives lack chromium, which is removed in the refining process. Chromium is needed for controlling blood sugar levels; when these levels are out of control it can trigger these behavioral problems.

7 A diet that is low in the essential nutrient calcium (needed to keep your bones strong) increases the risk of bones becoming weak or brittle – a condition known as osteoporosis.

8 A diet low in nutrients puts enormous strain on the liver. The liver is essential for the proper digestion and absorption of life-sustaining vitamins and minerals. For optimum health you need your liver to be in peak condition. The liver cannot cope with large amounts of saturated fat and alcohol and this can lead to liver and kidney problems, such as kidney disease and cirrhosis (a life-threatening condition where the cells of the liver die).

9 A diet too high in sugar can lead to too much glucose (a form of sugar carried in the bloodstream) circulating in your body. Too much glucose in the blood indicates development of blood sugar problems such as diabetes mellitus. Its symptoms are thirst, frequent need to urinate due to excess glucose, problems with vision, fatigue and recurrent infections.

10 If your diet is poor this can compromise your immune system and make you more susceptible to colds, flu and poor health. We need a steady and balanced intake of essential vitamins and minerals to keep our immune systems working properly, to provide protection from infections and disease.

10 FOODS PEOPLE EAT ON A REGULAR BASIS

This top 10 list of popular foods that many people eat on a regular basis may at first glance not appear too alarming, but just take a look at the nutritional analysis below. I have converted the statistics to teaspoons of sugar and sticks of butter to drum the facts home. Do you really still feel hungry?

1. Burger meal
2. Pizza
3. Spaghetti
4. Sweet 'n' sour pork with special fried rice (Chinese takeout)
5. Hot breakfast
6. Steak dinner
7. Nachos
8. Ice cream
9. Chocolate chip cookies
10. Hot dog meal

► **Burger meal (large burger, fries and cola)**
  - calories: 1300 ► protein: 34g
  - carbs: 189g fat: 44g ► fiber: 13g
  - equivalent to 38 teaspoons of sugar and ½ of a stick of butter

► **Pizza (medium deep pan pizza)**
  - calories: 1746 ► protein: 80g
  - carbs: 159g fat: 88g fiber: 8g
  - equivalent to 31 teaspoons of sugar and a stick of butter

► **Spaghetti (300g serving)**
  - calories: 237
  - carbs: 32g fat: 5.7g fiber: 3g
  - equivalent to 6 teaspoons of sugar

► **Chinese takeout (sweet 'n' sour pork with special fried rice)**
  - calories: 520 ► protein: 16g
  - carbs: 72g fat: 15g ► fiber: 1g
  - equivalent to 14 teaspoons of sugar and ⅙ of a stick of butter

► **Hot breakfast (2 scrambled eggs, 3 slices of bacon, pancakes, hash browns and a tall café latte with whole milk)**
  - calories: 1120 ► protein: 58g
  - carbs: 77g fat: 65.4g ► fiber: 2g
  - equivalent to 15 teaspoons of sugar and ¾ of a stick of butter

► **Steak dinner (8oz sirloin and baked potato with butter, sour cream and chives)**
calories: 994   protein: 73g
carbs: 60g   fat: 51.6g   fiber: 0g
equivalent to 12 teaspoons of sugar and ³/₅ of a stick of butter

► **Nachos (6 nacho chips smothered in cheese with chili, sour cream and guacamole)**
calories: 674   protein: 29g
carbs: 42g   fat: 44g   fiber: 2.5g
equivalent to 8 teaspoons of sugar and ½ of a stick of butter

► **Ice cream (chocolate, with chunks of brownies and walnuts)**
calories: 436   protein: 7.5g
carbs: 37.6g   fat: 28.6g   fiber: 0g
equivalent to 7 ½ teaspoons of sugar and ⅓ of a stick of butter

► **Chocolate chip cookies (8)**
calories: 636   protein: 7.6g
carbs: 76g   fat: 33g   fiber: 4.4g
equivalent to 15 teaspoons of sugar and nearly ³/₈ of a stick of butter

► **Hot dog meal (1 hot dog on a bun with ketchup, large fries and large Coke)**
calories: 1103   protein: 18g
carbs: 175g   fat: 35.6g   fiber: 8g
equivalent to 35 teaspoons of sugar and ²/₅ of a stick of butter

Now for the scary part: these are everyday foods that a lot of people consume regularly as part of their diet. What if you started your day with a lovely cooked breakfast, had a burger for lunch and went out for a pizza in the evening? (Don't forget I am not even counting snacks or drinks, just three meals.) Your totals would be:

calories: 3877   protein: 160g   carbs: 400g   fat: 182g   fiber: 31g

Normal daily average calorie intake is 2550 (17,850 per week) for men and 1940 (13,580 per week) for women. The above is almost double the recommended figure for women and over 1½ times for men.

It is the equivalent of eating twenty cotton candies a day and half of a block of lard. Start to add in the between-meal snacks, drinks, alcohol and not enough exercise and you become a ticking bomb of potential heart disease, diabetes, stroke, high blood pressure, digestive tract problems. Choose your poison – or as I hope, don't!

WHY DIETS DON'T WORK

Let's get something straight here. Conventional and traditional fad diets usually do not work. Calorie-counting diets, the "point system diet" or even the high-protein foods diet with no carbs – in my opinion these will all fail you and, even worse, most of them are tedious, pointless and downright dangerous to the body. Sure, they might help you to lose some weight in a few weeks or even in a few months. In the long run, though, you won't be able to continue with these fad diets because ultimately you will gain the weight back, and you won't be doing your body any favors.

Fad diets operate on restricting you, and in effect will usually starve you of something important that your body needs. For example, the extreme high-meat protein/low-carb diet craze is fundamentally, scientifically and nutritionally flawed. Every living human being must have complex carbohydrates to function, to think, for energy, for good sex and for a positive attitude. Complex carbohydrates include the important grains like brown rice, millet, quinoa, rye, barley and buckwheat. My patients who stopped eating complex carbohydrates for mostly high-protein foods started to seriously suffer from constipation, mood swings, anger fits, dizziness, headaches, stomach cramps and depression – even the most happy-go-lucky types. And in the long run, they had to come back to my lifestyle program for the most successful results.

In addition, most fad diets restrict the intake of essential fatty acids (EFAs). Again, this is bad science and it's bad for you too! EFAs actually help the body to dissolve fat. So to cut out foods high in them is like cutting out fat-burning agents. I call my program the Diet of Abundance, which is about *not* cutting out foods. Go on and eat those avocados, and those brazil nuts, almonds, sesame seeds, pumpkin seeds and walnuts, and the list goes on and on.

A "diet" to me is not about starving yourself, but rather a new lifestyle with an abundance of healthy foods. *You Are What You Eat* works better than anything else that has ever been tried, because my plan is based on scientific study from around the world, clinical research and biochemistry in the lab. Choose from a wonderful range of foods and embark upon the Dr. Gillian McKeith Lifestyle.

My aim is for you to make simple changes that will begin to take effect almost immediately and will last for life.

GOOD FOOD

These foods will:

- ► Boost your thinking power
- ► Lift your mood
- ► Reduce stress
- ► Boost your vitality
- ► Give you a healthier heart

When it comes to heart disease, a healthy diet is the prime player. It can:

- ► Supply chemicals in the blood that can unclog arteries, reduce cholesterol, create blood clot solvents and send hormones to relax artery walls, reducing blood pressure
- ► Play a part in the fight against cancer by releasing agents that can cause abnormal cell growths to shrink or disappear
- ► Help fight aging and slow down your body's natural deterioration
- ► Help chase away common colds and flu and stimulate your body to make more natural killer cells to ward off infection
- ► Prevent headaches and asthma attacks
- ► Create substances that can mute the pain and swelling of arthritis
- ► Attack bacteria and viruses
- ► Boost your fertility and sex drive
- ► Make your skin, hair and nails glow with health

There are countless other benefits, and it would be impossible to name them all. But my message here is loud and clear: **Healthy food choices can make you look and feel great.**

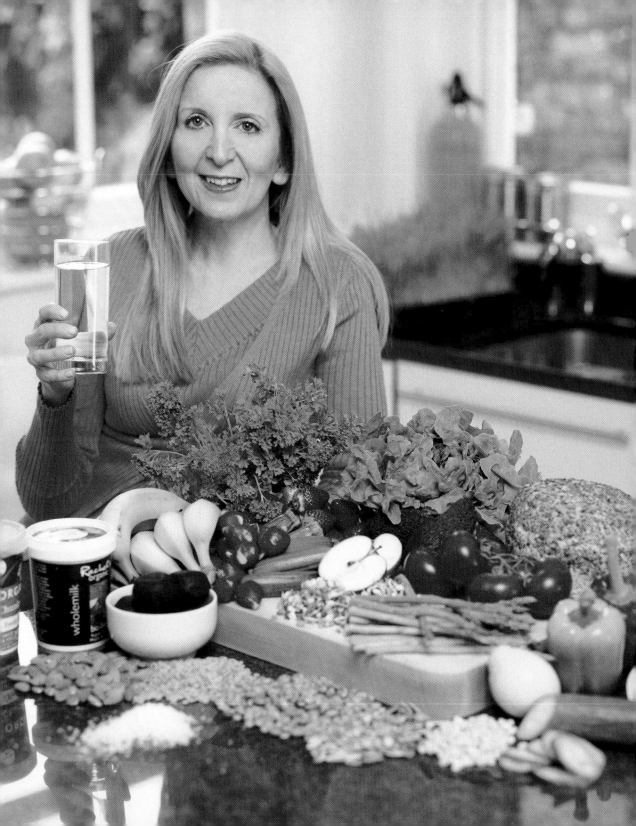

Basically if your diet isn't healthy, you won't feel healthy and you won't lose weight.

BAD FOOD

These foods will:
- Accelerate the aging process
- Cause weight gain
- Cause digestive problems, including bloating, gas and cramps
- Make you feel drowsy and lethargic
- Play havoc with your concentration
- Give you mood swings
- Adversely affect fertility and libido
- Set in process silent attacks that weaken the joints and clog the arteries, increasing the risk of heart disease and arthritis
- Make arteries narrow and stiff – just right for the formation of blood clots
- Promote toxic activity within the body that years later may end up as cancerous growth
- Weaken your immunity
- Trigger headaches and asthma attacks
- Increase the pain and swelling of arthritis
- Give you unhealthy-looking skin, hair and nails

GOOD FOOD V. BAD FOOD

GOOD FOOD

LIVING FOODS OR RAW FOODS

Living foods are raw foods. These foods have not been cooked, boiled, stewed, microwaved, frozen, baked or steamed. As a result, they are still in their original state and contain their food enzymes. Food enzymes are the life force of food and help the digestion process. Raw fruits, raw vegetables, sprouted grains or sprouted seeds all contain food enzymes. We need an abundant supply of food enzymes to nourish our bodies, provide us with energy and balance our metabolism.

The most noticeable deficit in my patients' old diets was that their meals were completely missing food enzymes. Most of them never ate anything raw.

GOOD CARBS

These are the carbs without the added refined sugar: for instance, fruits, whole grain breads, grains, rice and vegetables. These healthy carbohydrates (called complex carbs) contain naturally occurring sugars that the body can easily and slowly metabolize for balanced brain function, mood attitude and useful energy. They are not stripped of their nutrients.

ORGANIC FOODS

"Organic foods" means foods that are free of chemicals. Foods that are organic have been grown in soils that have not been sprayed with chemical fertilizers and pesticides. Remember, if chemicals have been sprayed on the produce that you eat, from chemically treated soils, then those chemicals, which are toxic, will enter your body cells and bloodstream. Who knows what damage they will do? There are numerous studies which show that chemicals inside our bodies do not help our health.

GOOD PROTEIN

Vegetable proteins are easy to break down in the body. Quinoa is an example of a vegetable protein that is very easy to digest. It looks like a grain and you can make a tasty porridge with it. Sprouts (not Brussels sprouts, but sprouts that are grown from seed) are a more efficient, cheaper and healthier form of protein than meat. Combining beans and grains together forms a complete protein too, easy to digest and enhancing to the metabolism.

GOOD FATS

Fats have a terrible reputation. In this era of low-fat foods and fat-free diets, the crusade against fats has almost gone mad. The most zealous campaigners even condemn oil-rich nutritious foods like nuts, seeds and avocados, but no one can ever blame heart disease on avocados!

I generally advocate good fat foods such as nuts, seeds and avocados to my patients. These oil-rich foods contain healthy fats which are necessary for aiding weight reduction, lowering cholesterol, enhancing immunity and nourishing the reproductive organs , skin, hair and bone tissue, effectively lubricating our bodies. These are the good fats, vitally important and necessary for life itself. And these fats help you to metabolize fat. They are so important that they are called essential fatty acids (EFAs).

Your body cannot make EFAs, so you must get them through the foods you eat. I think they really should be called essential thinny acids. That's how I refer to them in my practice and my patients seem to like the thinny concept better. Flax seeds, sunflower seeds, pumpkin seeds, sea vegetables, fish and avocados are good examples of these essential, thinny fats.

UNPROCESSED FOODS

These are foods that have no added chemicals or other additives. This food is in its orginal state, the way nature grew it. It has not been changed. Some packaged foods still contain foods and ingredients in their original state. Start reading labels (see page 176) and become more familiar with what goes into the foods you eat.

The crusade against fats has gone mad.

BAD FOOD

OVERCOOKED VEGGIES

Most of my patients, when they first come to see me, overcook vegetables. Many tell me they don't even like vegetables. I contend that they simply do not know how to prepare them. For some reason, we often have a tendency to boil our vegetables to death, and in the process lose all of their vital nutrients.

To get the most out of your veggies, either eat them raw or simply steam them lightly for two to three minutes maximum in most cases.

BAD CARBS

Simple carbs are the sugary, refined type of carbohydrates which are not good for you. These include chocolate, cakes, cookies, sweets and anything made with added, refined sugar or flour or processed white rice. During the refining process, the majority of the minerals and vitamins are removed, and these foods behave like pure sugar when they enter the body. They rush into the bloodstream, causing blood glucose disturbances and sugar cravings. Eat too many of these foods and you will undoubtedly have mood swings. You may get depressed, angry and irritable. If you want to be fat and ill, eat bad carbs. Excess bad carb residues are stored as fat in the body. And finally, years of bad carb eating could lead to diabetes. It's not worth the risk.

NON-ORGANIC FOODS

Non-organic foods, such as non-organic fruits and vegetables, have been sprayed with chemicals and grown in soils that have been treated with chemical fertilizers and pesticides. The residues of these chemicals make their way into our bodies when we eat these non-organic foods. They harm our cells and organs and damage our digestive systems. These chemicals become toxins in our bodies, polluting and poisoning us.

BAD PROTEIN

Depending on how strong your digestive system is, some proteins may simply not be good enough for you. Most people on my TV show *You Are What You Eat* had very weak digestive function, so proteins from red meats were hard for them to break down.

Too many high-protein, fatty, red animal foods can toxify the body and acidify the blood, deplete calcium, overwork the kidneys and liver, stagnate digestion and destroy the beneficial bacteria. This can also lead to kidney stones and liver fatigue, colon and bowel disorders, constipation, arthritis, osteoporosis and heart disease.

Even cow's milk is too difficult for many people to digest. It can trigger allergic responses such as sinusitis, asthma, earache, congestion, runny nose, skin rash, eczema, fatigue, lethargy and irritability. Whole cow's milk is too high in saturated fat, low in vitamins, and the mineral content is out of balance with human biochemistry; as a result, many of the nutrients cannot be absorbed by humans. Also, cows are normally subjected to hundreds of different drug injections, hormones, pesticides, drug residues which in turn make their way into the milk. If you must drink cow's milk, boil it first to make it easier to digest.

Try goat and sheep's milk as alternatives, as the molecules are smaller and easier to break down. There is also an abundance of alternative milks on the market that are easy to digest: rice milks, soy milks and other grain milks.

REFINED FOODS

The modern diet contains many refined foods. All the participants on *You Are What You Eat* had diets full of refined foods. Refined foods are stripped of their original, natural nutrient content and fiber. The consumer is left with a more concentrated, unnatural sweet version of the original food. Refined white flour and white sugar are the two most common examples of refined foods. These ingredients are then used in a multitude of other "foods." Baked goods, chocolates, fast foods and frozen dinners to name a few are the types of foods filled with additives and preservatives to give them a longer shelf life. These foods really should be called "non-foods." They cause havoc with the health of the body as the body is not designed to deal with these nutrient-depleted, industrial, false foods.

On the show, I met one participant who only ate refined, processed, preservative-laden foods. Yvonne, who was overweight, depressed, exhausted and constipated, survived mainly on chips and microwaved meals. She never, ever ate real food. To bring Yvonne to her senses, I teasingly suggested that if she were to drop dead tomorrow, her body would literally take years to decompose because she was so full of all these preservatives. That was a bit of a shock, but she definitely got the message!

BAD FATS

Saturated animal fats are heavy and turn to stone inside the body, hardening the arteries, leaving you at risk of heart attack and stroke. Red meat, pork, dairy products, butter and cheese are examples of foods that are fat saturated. The body is not designed to deal with these types of fats. High bad-fat diets raise blood pressure and cholesterol levels, can interfere with blood sugar levels and cause liver stagnation, which can lead to depression and weight gain. The body cannot effectively process bad fats, so many are turned into toxic balls and stored in the body, making you even fatter.

Hydrogenated fats are the results of a process that hardens liquid vegetable oils. Shortening and margarine are hydrogenated fats, so potato chips, chocolate, sweets, ice cream, pastries and baked goods all contain hydrogenated fats. The hydrogenated fats change into the ever more dangerous trans-fatty acids which have been shown to cause diabetes, heart disease and cancer. Trans-fatty acids also cause you to gain weight as they interfere with the metabolism and breakdown of essential fatty acids. They increase the bad cholesterol in the body and deplete the good.

PROCESSED FOODS

The processing of foods changes the original food and the proportions of the nutrients within these foods. Many prepackaged and plastic-wrapped foods, quick fix, microwaveable, fast and boil-in-the-bag type foods have gone through a multitude of processes before they end up in the supermarket. These foods have little or no nutritional value.

The food industry allows more than three thousand food additives to be used in the processing of food. And just because many of these additives and chemicals used in the processing of our foods are deemed safe, it does not mean that they are. So chemicals, food additives, coloring agents, sweeteners, artificial flavors, dyes, nitrates, nitrites, preservatives to prevent spoilage, acids, maturing agents, bleaching agents, emulsifiers to maintain consistency are all finding their way into our bodies via these easy-to-prepare packaged foods.

These processes can cause allergic reactions and stress on the liver to process such chemicals, many of which are cancer forming. Children exposed to such processes can become hyperactive and display learning difficulties.

THE WORST EATER I EVER MET

Andy, a twenty-six-year-old computer specialist from Essex, England, took part in the pilot for the TV show *You Are What You Eat*. His girlfriend had just left him a week before and it had been a terrible shock. He was devastated and severely depressed when I first met him.

Andy's life consisted of gorging on food during the day and bingeing on drink at the pub in the evening. A sample of his everyday diet: potato chips, chocolate, white bread, burgers, more burgers and even more burgers, French fries and loads of beer. This young, blond, strapping six-foot two-inch man with chiseled features weighed 392 pounds. Andy was clinically obese and his poor food choices were ruining his life. He was exhausted, out of breath, had terrible indigestion, gas and bloating, and was really down in the dumps. His gooey, sticky, slimy, unhealthy stools stank to high heaven and he was sweating far too much, even when sitting down.

My biochemical tests revealed that his mineral and vitamin profiles were dreadful and he had the lowest level of essential fatty acids (EFAs) I have ever seen in my many years of practice. This meant he could not break down fats properly.

I gave him an ultimatum: Follow my program or die young. Do what I tell you and I will continue to work with you. Step out of line and I walk out on you. Andy made the right choice. He wholeheartedly embarked upon my program, which was as follows:

- No red meat
- No refined white sugar
- No refined floury pastries
- No chips or fries
- No alcohol
- Unlimited amounts of fresh raw fruits and vegetables, raw seeds, nuts and some legumes, pulses and grains
- Moderate daily exercise

This pub-crawling greaser even started to juice his own wheatgrass and carrot juices every day, instead of downing pints at his local. End result: Andy lost over fifty-six pounds in less than three months and he felt great. Although he is still in the process of losing additional fat, today Andy is a new man and he looks great too.

GOOD FOOD = BETTER LIFE

So you can see how food makes all the difference to your health and well-being. It provides the great majority of the nutrients you need to stay healthy and happy. Food has the most incredible influence on your emotional, mental and physical states. Eating healthy, high-quality food is one of the easiest and most powerful ways to create a better life. By thinking more closely about what you eat and making healthier food choices, you can get the most of your food and the best out of your life. Because you truly are what you eat!

CHAPTER 2

GET TO KNOW YOUR BODY

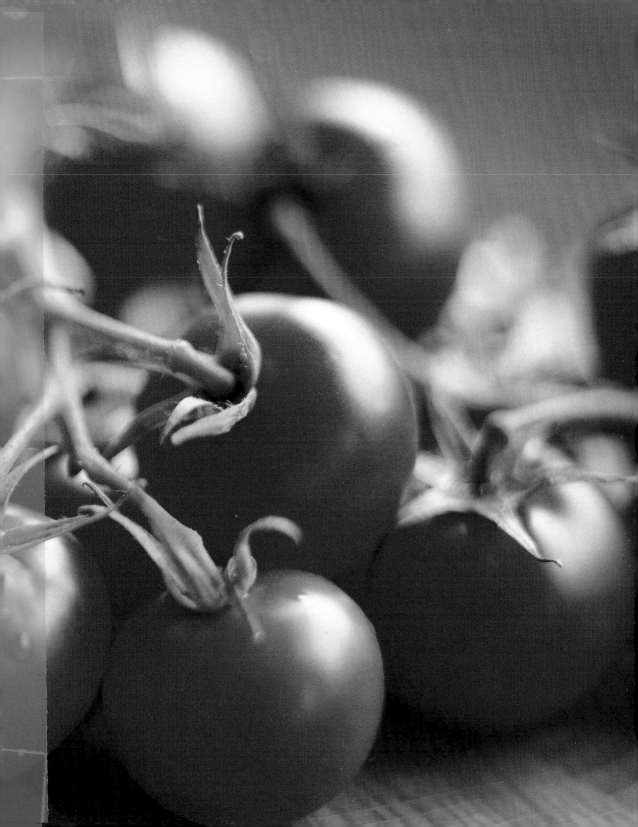

Joanne, a cuddly mother of three, just couldn't stop eating. She had tried to lose weight many times on many fad diets but to no avail. She told me that she was too tired to even take her sons to the park and just wanted to sleep and eat. Her daily routine was based on what, where and when she would eat next, but she longed to feel good about herself again.

Joanne consumed the equivalent of 664 teaspoons of white, processed sugar in a week and 1173 grams in fat, which is equal to 4½ blocks of pig lard. She lived on a diet of junk food, bacon and eggs, burgers, chocolate and two liters of soda every day. There was nothing fresh or raw in her food intake. Weighing in at 322 pounds, twenty-nine-year-old Joanne was depressed, her gums bled, she had poor memory, no energy, absolutely no sex drive, bad breath, mood swings, hair loss and hideous cellulite. She bloated like a balloon after eating anything and was full of gas. She suffered daily headaches and lived on painkillers.

Joanne had no knowledge of the ravaging effects that white, processed sugar and saturated fats could have on the body. These types of foods were what she was raised on; she continued to eat this way and fed her kids the same diet too.

Twenty-eight-year-old Julie, mom to a four-year-old girl, was a migraine sufferer and was seriously constipated to the point that she could only move her bowels once a week if she took laxatives. She had hemorrhoids, problems sleeping, acne, bleeding gums, menstrual cramps similar to labor pains, gas and no stamina or energy.

Both Joanne and Julia had to go through my body check consultation, where I check tongues, nails and other body signs. Joanne's tongue was loaded with cuts, serrations, peelings, raised sore areas and dirty coatings.

All of this indicated deficiencies of vital nutrients needed for weight management and a healthy functioning body. I could see from her tongue that she was loaded with nasty bacterias, her body wasn't able to deal with the vast amount of saturated bad fats she was forcing it to process, her organs were functioning under par, and I could predict various health ailments from which she must be suffering. Joanne was indeed stunned by my accurate predictions, which I made simply by reading her tongue.

Joanne's fingernails were bitten down to the quick, another sign of mineral depletions. She had to be exhausted. Her body was eating itself in a desperate bid for minerals. She was certainly not getting them from her beefburger diet.

Julie's tongue showed a great deal too. Most revealing was her stomach, intestines and lung function. I could tell that her tummy was weak, digestion abominable, that her intestines were clogged with old matter and her lungs had been damaged from years of smoking. She had cuts on the sides and in the middle of her tongue, indicating nutrient imbalances and chronic deficiencies.

When I laid both girls down on the floor and gently felt their stomachs and the area below the right rib, the site of the liver, Joanne almost went through the roof and Julie gasped at the sharpness of her pain. These pain reactions are not normal and a sign that all is not well. Both girls were toxic, inflamed and harboring poisons. Their diets were destroying them. Their bodies were screaming for help.

Sometimes you don't need to go to a nutritionist to find out what's wrong with your diet. There are some very easy signs to look for on your own body that can tell you – it's all a matter of being body aware.

THE TOP BODY SIGNS

Here are the *most common* body signs to look out for to assess the state of your health. Each one is followed by information on what it means, plus pointers on what to do about it. Follow them and you're on a surefire path to good health.

Artichokes
Avocados
Carrots
Millet sprouts
Parsnips
Rice
Squash
Sweet potatoes
Tofu
Turnips
Yams
Teas/herbs:
fennel,
peppermint,
licorice

THE TONGUE

The tongue is an important indicator of health so I'd like to start by focusing on it in some detail.

I always think of the tongue as being like a window to the organs. The extreme tip correlates to the heart, the bit slightly behind is the lungs. The right side shows what the gallbladder is up to and the left side the liver. The middle indicates the condition of your stomach and spleen, the back the kidneys, intestines, bladder and womb.

A healthy tongue should be smooth, supple and slightly moist. It should be pale red in color with a very thin, white film. The most common tongue indicators I look out for are cracks, ravines, coatings (e.g., yellow/ furry/ thick/ white), lines, swellings, patches of red and cuts.

CRACK DOWN THE MIDDLE

A midline crack not reaching the tip seems harmless enough but if you have one, it means you have a weak stomach and your digestion is not what it should be. You are most likely nutrient-depleted. And I bet you are often bloated after eating and maybe even a victim of energy slumps in the middle of the day, especially after lunch. You are certainly not as energized as you could be. But then again, most people have no idea how well they could really be.

Solutions:

▸ Learn how to food combine – this means avoiding eating certain food groups at the same time (see page 78).

▸ Take a digestive enzyme with meals – this is a supplement which helps to break down food during digestion (see page 209).

▸ Eat soups, stews and blends – foods that are easy to digest. Millet porridge would be good for you.

▸ Don't guzzle fizzy drinks and don't drink liquids at mealtimes.

▸ See *Foods to Nourish the Tummy*, above.

The spleen is a small organ that has many functions. It works in tandem with your stomach for the uptake of nutrients from the foods you eat and is responsible for getting rid of worn-out red blood cells by recycling them and transforming them into iron to build the blood. It also neutralizes unhealthy bacteria, so helps prevent colds and flu when it is strong. Yours is not doing this effectively if you have teethmarks around the side of your tongue.

Garlic
Black pepper
Ginger
Cayenne pepper
Ginseng
Cinnamon
Horseradish
Dill seed
Pau d'arco
Astragalus

TEETHMARKS AROUND THE SIDES

Teethmarks around the sides of the tongue are a sign of nutritional deficiency. The likelihood is that your digestion is also impaired and you have a spleen deficiency.

Sluggish spleen function is very common. Around 70 percent of the patients I meet for the first time suffer from it. If your spleen is weak, you probably put up with gas and bloating.

Solutions:
Eat foods which nourish the spleen:

- Aduki beans
- Yellow squash
- Mung beans
- Kidney beans
- Alfalfa
- Lychees
- Barley
- Millet
- Beetroot
- Oats
- Carrots
- Parsley
- Celery
- Parsnips
- Chicken

- Pumpkin
- Fennel
- Root vegetables
- Fish
- Sweet potatoes
- Turnips
- Yams

Foods high in chlorophyll:

- Leafy greens
- Algae
- Kale
- Chard

SORE TONGUE

A sore tongue is a sure sign of a nutrient deficiency – often iron, vitamin B6 or niacin.

Solutions:

- Take liquid mineral supplements and start to drink nettle teas, which are high in these much-needed minerals.
- Get your iron levels checked. Iron deficiency can sometimes be caused by vitamin B12, folic acid or copper deficiencies. See a nutritionist for advice.

BURNING TONGUE

A sign that the stomach is lacking in gastric digestive juices. You may also experience tummy trouble if you have this symptom.

Solutions:

- Try taking a teaspoon of Swedish Bitters daily. It will really help to increase your gastric juice secretions.
- Drink a cup of dandelion tea twice a day.
- Take a teaspoon of apple cider vinegar before each meal.
- HCL (hydrochloric acid) tablets can help to adjust the gastric juices in the stomach.

SWOLLEN TONGUE AND/ OR THICK WHITE COATING

These are indicators that there is too much mucus in the body. They are also signs of a lack of beneficial bacteria and also, possibly, an elevation of yeasts.

Solutions:

▶ Cut down on dairy products. These foods are mucus-producing and your inner organs are too damp to deal with them.

▶ Read the section on superfoods (see page 200). Introduce one green superfood into your life.

▶ See page 76 to read about yeast control.

▶ Get acidophilus powder or capsules from a health store to replenish your body with healthy bacteria. You will need a six-month course.

▶ Drink pau d'arco tea (pronounced *poh darko*), available from health stores. This is a superb way to lower the yeasts in your body.

▶ The homeopathic remedy Bryonia (available from health food shops) may help, especially if your mouth is dry and you are quite thirsty.

HORIZONTAL CRACKS, SMALL CRACKS/GROOVES

Sometimes referred to as a geographic tongue. Cracking on the tongue is a sign of malabsorption, especially of B vitamins, and is often accompanied by a lack of energy. Most overweight patients I see for the first time are deficient in this vital nutrient. The deficiency is likely to have been over a lengthy period of time – cracks like this take a long time to develop.

Solutions:

▶ Add vitamin B Complex (50mg a day) to your diet.

▶ Take a digestive enzyme supplement with meals (see page 209).

▶ Change your diet to include foods that are high in food enzymes and easier to absorb (see page 209)

▶ Take echinacea tincture (20 drops daily for two weeks) – to help move lymph and eliminate toxins that are impeding nutrient absorption.

▶ Drink slippery elm or peppermint teas to help calm the stomach.

▶ Nettle tea will help fortify the body with B vitamins.

▶ Drink 2 tablespoons of aloe vera juice before meals.

A red tip on your tongue could indicate a recent emotional upset.

THICK YELLOW COATING

A thick yellow coating on the tongue indicates excess heat in the gut. It also means you don't have enough healthy bacteria in your body. If the coating is at the back of the tongue, you need to pay attention to your colon. Your bowels are not working as well as they should be.

Solutions:

► You may be run down from doing too much, so start to take things easier.
► Cool yourself down with 2 tablespoons of aloe vera juice before meals.
► Start eating the foods in Chapter 3, "The Diet of Abundance," and these problems should ease.
► Drink sage tea (2 cups a day for a month). Alternate with camomile tea.

RED TIP

A red tip on the tongue indicates emotional upset or emotional stress. It could be something from the past that you are still unconsciously holding on to, or due to present circumstances. A red tip on the tongue can also indicate emotional strain in your body.

Emotional upset disturbs the normal energy balance within the body, causing your inner energy to stagnate, especially if the strain is prolonged. You may have an excess of stress hormones flowing through your system.

Some people are better than others at dealing with upset. A young woman in her early thirties once came to see me. When I looked at her tongue, I noticed a very red tip so I asked her if she had experienced any emotional upheavals in her life. She quickly snapped back that she hadn't. But about five minutes later, she burst into tears and explained that she had just broken up with her boyfriend of seven years and was heartbroken. It showed . . . on her tongue.

Solutions:

► See page 113 on how to deal with stress.
► The herbs Siberian ginseng and rhodiola – both available from health food stores – are helpful for stress.

HEAD

DANDRUFF ON THE SCALP

This can be due to yeast overgrowth and/or deficiencies of EFAs, vitamin B6 and/or selenium.

Solutions:

- Take 2 tablespoons of flax oil a day.
- Take the antifungal herb pau d'arco, either in the form of tea (2 cups a day) or capsules (3, taken twice a day) and immediately reduce the amount of sugary foods you eat.
- Eat foods high in food enzymes (see page 209).
- Add the following hair-nourishing supplements to your diet every day: selenium (200mcg), biotin (600mcg), and 1 Reishi mushroom capsule.
- Wash your hair with camomile or tea tree shampoos. After washing, rinse with 1 cup of cider vinegar and 10 drops of peppermint oil.

FACE

VEINS CLOSE TO SURFACE ON CHEEKS/RAISED CAPILLARIES

A sign of digestive enzyme insufficiency or low stomach acid.

Solutions:

- Take HCL supplements (1 tablet before your largest meal of the day) and a digestive enzyme supplement, taken with a sip of water halfway through the meal. One tablespoon of apple cider vinegar before meals can help too.
- Be aware that your body is screaming for food enzymes (see page 209). You need to eat more sprouted seeds, sprouted grains, raw fruits and raw veggies.

EARS

CRACKS BEHIND THE EARS

Cracks behind the ears are a sign of a zinc deficiency. Zinc deficiencies can take a long time to correct – at least six months to a year.

Solution:

- ► Start with 1 teaspoon of liquid zinc supplement mixed in juice daily, then move on to zinc citrate capsules (25mg a day).
- ► Eat pumpkin seeds, sesame seeds and papayas.

WAX OOZING FROM THE EARS

You have an EFA deficiency – a very common problem in this country. Too many people avoid fats in an effort to lose weight. The mistake they make is they avoid good fats as well as bad. Then, when they want a treat, they usually opt for the bad fat treat instead of the good.

Solutions:

- ► Drizzle 2 tablespoons of flax oil or linseeds over your salads.
- ► Take extra evening primrose oil, borage oil, omega-3 or SLA (1000mg a day).
- ► Cut down on cow's milk products.

HANDS

BREAKING/SPLITTING/ CHIPPING NAILS

These are an indication that your liver needs help. They may also be a sign of calcium, zinc or EFA deficiencies, or low stomach acid.

Solutions:

► Take the herb milk thistle (2 capsules a day).

► Eat broccoli, Brussels sprouts, cabbage, whole grains, amaranth, chicory, all kinds of seeds and the sea vegetable nori.

► Drink 2 cups of nettle tea a day. Nettle tea is a panacea for delivering nutrients to the body. I love it.

WHITE SPOTS

White spots on the nails are a classic sign of zinc deficiency. More than 80 percent of the people who come to see me test zinc-deficient. By the time the white spots reach your nails, your zinc levels are pretty low, and you need to do something about it soon.

Solutions:

► Start taking 1 teaspoon of liquid algae and 1 tablet of zinc supplement daily.

► Snack on pumpkin seeds and sunflower seeds for their zinc content.

CRACKS ON THE SKIN/TINY BLISTERS ON THE FINGERTIPS

A sign of zinc deficiency.

Solution:

► See Solutions, above, for White Spots.

SWOLLEN FINGERS OR PUFFY HANDS

A sign of B6 deficiency.

Solutions:

► Eat plenty of food high in B vitamins, such as brown rice, sunflower seeds, avocados, buckwheat and legumes.

► You may need an additional daily dose of 35mg B6.

► Drink red clover tea (3 cups a day).

RED, SCALY SKIN ON HANDS

You could have zinc, EFA, vitamin C and E deficiencies. Red, scaly skin can also be a sign of food sensitivities.

Solutions:

► Try adding 25mg zinc, 1000mg EFAs, 1000mg vitamin C and 400iu vitamin E to your daily diet.

► Get yourself tested for food sensitivities (see page 96). You could start by eradicating the most likely suspects: wheat and chocolate.

EYES

PALE INSIDE LOWER EYELID

Pull the lower eyelid down. Inside the lower rim, the color should be pinky red. If it's extremely pale, you may be anemic. You may need iron plus vitamin B complex with B12.

Solutions:

► Get this checked by your GP or a specialist nutritionist.

► Start taking a liquid mineral supplement following the dosage on the packaging, or daily multivitamin/mineral supplement.

► Nettle tea is a great natural iron booster.

DARK CIRCLES UNDER THE EYES

Dark circles under the eyes usually indicate food allergies and possible weak kidney energy.

Solutions:

► Rotate your foods; in other words, do not eat the same foods every day.

► Eat the grain quinoa (see page 212).

► Drink cranberry juice (2 glasses daily for a week).

► Build up your kidneys by eating the foods listed below:

FOODS TO NOURISH THE KIDNEYS

GRAINS	BEANS	FISH	LEGUMES
Barley	Aduki beans	Salmon	Mung beans
Quinoa	Black beans	Trout	Water chestnuts
Wheat berries	Kidney beans		Black sesame seeds
Sweet rice			Walnuts

HERBS/TEAS	VEGETABLES	FRUITS	SUPPLEMENTS
Cloves	Fennel	Blackberries	Magnesium
Cinnamon bark	Onions	Blueberries	(300mg, twice a day)
Fenugreek	Spring onions		Horsetail
Garlic	Chives		(500mg, twice a day)
Ginger	Beetroot		
Raspberry	Parsley	SUPERFOODS	
Blackberry	Celery	Seaweeds	
Schisandra		Chlorella	
Gravel root			
Rose hips			
Dandelion			
Uva ursi (or in capsule form 500mg)			

MOUTH

CRACKS AT EACH CORNER OF THE MOUTH

A sign of vitamin B2 deficiency.

Solutions:

► Drink 2 cups of red clover/nettle tea every day.
► Take a vitamin B complex supplement that contains B2 (riboflavin) (50mg daily).
► Drink a glass of carrot juice with a teaspoon of the superfood spirulina every day.
► Eat plenty of dark green leafy veggies, almonds, parsley and wheat germ.

PUFFY LOWER LIP

Unless you've been injected with collagen to give your lips a fuller appearance, a puffy lower lip indicates digestive stagnation. It could even suggest constipation. Bear in mind that even if you move your bowels every day, it does not mean you are not constipated. Not everything we eat comes out as effectively as it should!

Solutions:

► Eat simply, food combine (see page 78), drink warm herbal teas and eat hearty vegetable soups.
► A digestive enzyme supplement along with the superfood spirulina should make a difference.
► Slippery elm tea will soothe your system.

LIMBS

TENDER SPOTS WHERE THE SHOULDER MEETS YOUR ARM

An indication of vitamin B12 deficiency.

Solution:

► Get B12 sublingual lozenges from a health store (1000mcg daily).

SMALL PIMPLY BUMPS ON THE ARM

A possible sign of beta-carotene, B complex and EFA deficiency.

Solutions:

► Take the above supplements (beta-carotene 15mg daily, B complex 50mg daily and EFA 500mcg daily).
► Take digestive enzymes to help you absorb other nutrients.
► Start eating a wide range of foods which contain high levels of B12, including sprouted seeds, fish, tempeh, miso soup and dulse.

Deficiencies of the mineral magnesium are at epidemic levels in the U.S., causing constipation, high blood pressure, depression, leg cramps, PMS, insomnia and excessive tiredness.

RED SPOTS ON THE FRONT OF THE THIGH

A possible vitamin A deficiency.

Solutions:

► Take wild blue-green algae supplement (6 tablets or 1 teaspoon daily) or the superfood spirulina in powder form or tablets (1 teaspoon daily or 6 tablets).

► Add seaweed to your cooking (see page 208).

► Take a good multivitamin supplement daily.

► Try an additional supplement of beta-carotene (15mg daily) – it sounds strange but it's a very good source of vitamin A.

► Eat plenty of foods from the following list, all high in vitamin A:

► Broccoli
► Brussels sprouts
► Carrots
► Dandelion greens
► Halibut
► Kale
► Mustard green
► Papaya
► Parsley
► Pumpkin
► Red pepper
► Salmon
► Sweet potatoes
► Watermelon
► Watercress
► Yellow squash

SORE KNEE

If your knee is sore where the kneecap joins the main bone of the leg, it could be an indicator of vitamin and mineral deficiencies.

Solution:

► Try 400mcg selenium and vitamin E for two to three months.

SORE LOWER LEG BONE

A lower leg bone that is sore when pressed is an indicator of vitamin and mineral deficiency.

Solution:

► Take calcium (1000mg daily) and niacinimide (500mcg daily).

LEG CRAMPS

Cramping leg pain means your calcium levels are low. You may also have a magnesium deficiency, since magnesium is needed to mobilize calcium into the bones.

Solutions:

► Take 750mg magnesium and 500mg calcium twice a day.

► Add seaweed to your soups and stews.

► Eat lots of green leafy vegetables.

► If you exercise often and sweat, it's a good idea to take a magnesium supplement after your workout.

VARICOSE VEINS

An indication of nutritional deficiencies and/or congestion in the liver.

Solutions:

► Take vitamin E (400iu daily), bioflavanoids (500mg daily) and magnesium (1000mg daily).

► See page 49 for my 10-Point Hemorrhoid Plan. Follow this advice and you will help your varicose veins too! See also page 162.

CRACKED FEET

Cracking on your feet indicates a possible rise of yeast in the body.

Solutions:

► Add a biotin supplement to your diet (50mg daily) to prevent yeast organisms from budding full cycle.

► Massage your feet with flax oil.

STOMACH

TENDER, GASSY STOMACH THAT IS SOMETIMES PAINFUL

An indication of low stomach acid and insufficient digestive enzymes.

Solutions:

► Take an HCL supplement.

► Take a digestive enzyme with each meal.

► Cut out cow's milk products, because the molecules are too large for many people to break down in the stomach.

► Try food combining (see page 78).

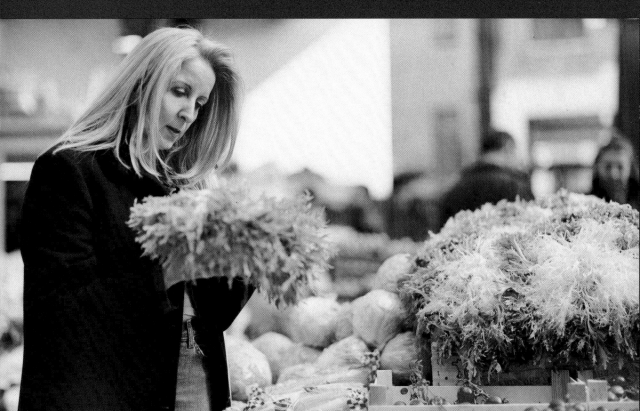

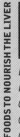

Broccoli
Brussels sprouts
Cabbage
Cauliflower
Garlic
Eggs
Kohlrabi
Turnip roots
Nuts
Seeds
(especially flax,
sunflower and
pumpkin)

STOOLS

GREASY STOOLS THAT WON'T FLUSH
Floating stools that will not flush show a liver imbalance.
Solutions:
▶ Start sprinkling linseeds on your salads or into soups every day.
▶ Practice the Liver Rub (see page 150).
▶ Drink 3 cups of sage tea a day.
▶ Take a teaspoon of spirulina every day.
▶ Eat more of the foods in the list (left) to strengthen the liver.
▶ Take L-Glutamine powder before all meals (see page 108).
▶ Cleanse your body out with the ayurvedic cleansing tri herb combination Triphala. If you can't find that anywhere, get psyllium husks and treat yourself to a home enema (see page 151).

FOUL-SMELLING STOOLS
Foul-smelling stools are a sign of poor digestion and food stagnating in your large intestine. This means you are toxic and your gut is overly acidic. You are sorely in need of digestive enzymes.
Solutions:
▶ Start taking a digestive enzyme capsule with every meal.
▶ Buy some liquid chlorophyll from a health food store and take a teaspoon before meals.
▶ Take 100mg coenzyme Q10 every day.
▶ It would do you the world of good to start juicing your own juice (for example, 2 carrots, 2 sticks of celery and 1 cucumber, juiced together). I know that sounds like a pain but it's well worth the bother.

SKID MARK STOOLS

Your stools have too much mucus, so they slide and stick to the edge of the toilet. You are lacking good-quality fiber in your diet and need to eat more foods high in food enzymes (see page 209). The stickiness is a sign of dampness inside the body – a very common condition.

Solutions:

▸ Reduce your intake of mucus-producing foods such as dairy products and alcohol. Yep. Skip the pub visits for a while or stick to still mineral water. I am not trying to be a party pooper but you will feel miles better within just a few days.

▸ Eat the superfood wild blue-green algae, available from health food stores (6 capsules a day). See page 204.

PELLETS

If you are producing rabbit droppings, then your liver needs help as it is congested. I urge my own patients at the clinic to embark upon my one-day detox (see page 140) but I make them do it for two days!

Solutions:

▸ Take 2 capsules of milk thistle, three times a day, and alpha lipoic acid (500mg daily) for a month.

▸ Use an internal cleansing powder called psyllium or Triphala (2 tablespoons mixed in juice or water a day) and take 1 teaspoon liquid chlorophyll before meals. You can get all of this in a health store.

▸ Sprinkle 2 tablespoons of lecithin granules on cereals or salads.

LIGHT-COLORED STOOLS

If your stools are light beige in color or have a yellow appearance it's a sign that you have difficulty digesting fatty foods. You are also most likely deficient in essential fatty acids, the good fats.

Solutions:

▸ Eat more foods with EFAs, to help you to metabolize fats. Add fish, avocados, pumpkin seeds, sunflower seeds and sea vegetables such as nori and dulse to your diet.

▸ Sprinkling 1 tablespoon of flax seeds over salad will also help normalize your stools.

FOOD IN YOUR STOOLS

It is normal to find sweetcorn skin in your stools as the outer skin is fairly indigestible. However, if you find remnants of other foods, then it may mean your digestive system is weak. Also, you may not be chewing your food enough. Chew your food thoroughly and remember that your stomach doesn't have any teeth.

WORMS IN YOUR STOOLS

A horrible thought, but it's more widespread than you can imagine. Children often have them and pass them on to adults through poor hygiene. You can also pick them up from kissing your pets on the mouth, eating poorly cooked pork, raw meats or raw fish.

Deworm yourself right away. If you have worms, you will be low in nutrients. The worms are living off your nutrients and your nutrient absorption will be compromised. People with worms often have anemia (low iron levels). Get your iron levels checked out.

You will most likely have a very itchy bottom, especially at night. Try not to scratch as they can spread this way.

Solutions:

The following can help and may sound alien to you but they work. It means making a trip to the health food store for some of the items but it's worth it:

► Black walnut tincture destroys worms. Take it three times daily on an empty stomach. A combination of cloves, wormwood and black walnut tincture works best, but don't take this combination if you are pregnant.

► Gentiana root tincture, three times daily, is superb for treating worms.

► Eat lots of pumpkin seeds, sesame seeds and figs to expel the little creatures.

► Drink aloe vera juice one or two times a day before meals to help prevent reinfection.

► Take a good multivitamin with high levels of B vitamins.

► Grapefruit seed extract (20 drops in water three times a day) is a good natural remedy.

► Eat lots of onions, dark green leafy vegetables and salads.

► Cut out sweets, pasteurized milks and processed foods. Worms thrive in that environment.

► Drink senna tea to pump out those little creatures.

► Zinc oxide cream smoothed on the opening of the anus will help relieve discomfort.

► It may sound crazy, but put a couple of garlic cloves inside your socks/shoes. As you walk, the garlic will be crushed up and will absorb through your skin into the blood to the intestinal tract. Worms hate garlic and you absorb the antiparasitic properties through your skin. Of course, eating raw or cooked garlic would work too!

LOOSE AND RUNNY STOOLS ALL THE TIME

This is not the same as a single bout of diarrhea caused by a bug. This is a situation whereby you are always having runny stools that are never formed. It's a sign that your spleen function is exhausted (see page 34).

Solutions:

► This is the one time where I would not encourage you to eat too many raw veggies until your stools have improved.
► Add the following to your diet: onions, leeks, ginger, cinnamon, fennel, garlic and nutmeg.
► Rice, oats and spelt are great breakfast starters for this condition.
► See page 34 for list of foods beneficial to the spleen.
► Take acidophilus supplements (follow dosage instructions on the package).
► Eat warm foods and drink herbal teas or warm water, especially during cold or rainy months. If you want to eat salads, always have a warm food with them, or grate ginger over the salad. Grated ginger will have a warming effect on the spleen.

THIN, SHREDDY STOOLS

Your colon is screaming out for help. Please clean me!

Solutions:

► Giving yourself an enema or having colonic irrigation would be a good idea (see page 151).
► Eat a diet high in fiber, i.e., lots of fruits, vegetables and dark green leafy salads.
► Go on my one-day detox (see page 140) for more than one day!
► Get psyllium husks or Triphala and follow the directions on the label.

Top Tip: How much time?
If you want to see how long you are taking to digest your veggies, then eating corn is one way to find out. From the moment the corn enters your mouth until it reaches your stools, the process should take about six hours. Any longer and your digestion is not as efficient as it should be. If it is taking longer try drinking two tablespoons of aloe vera juice before meals and a digestive enzyme supplement with all meals to help break down your foods.

ITCHY BOTTOM

Don't feel embarrassed about this one. Loads of people have itchy bottoms. This usually indicates one of the following three conditions: worms or parasites (see page 45), food sensitivities or hemorrhoids. Please be fastidious about hand washing.

FOOD SENSITIVITIES

To check out if this is the case, try the Food Sensitivity Pulse Test below. The average pulse rate is fairly even, but when you eat foods to which you may be sensitive, your heartbeat increases. Do the test and if your pulse changes after eating a meal, you may have food sensitivities. All you need is a watch with a second hand.

PULSE TEST METHOD

► First thing in the morning when you wake up, take your radial pulse. Place your pointer finger on the radial pulse (on your wrist). Count the number of beats in a 60-second period. Your reading should be somewhere between 50 and 70 beats per 60 seconds.

► After eating a meal, take your radial pulse again. If the pulse reading score has increased by more than 10 beats, then you may have a sensitivity to a particular food within the meal. You will then need to separate out the foods to find the one to which you are reacting, using the same method outlined above.

Solutions:

► Take 1 teaspoon of L-Glutamine powder before meals to help minimize food reactions.

► Eggs, citrus fruits, soya products, corn, wheat, dairy products, tomatoes and spicy foods can often aggravate the problem. Avoid them where possible.

HEMORRHOIDS

When your liver is congested, you usually end up with hemorrhoids. Hemorrhoids are swollen bluish, reddish or purple, often large, inflamed veins and capillaries around the anus. They appear in various sizes generally from the size of a pea to the size of a grapefruit. They can be seriously uncomfortable. You will congest your liver through poor food choices. Too much sugar, chocolate, coffee, cream, pastries, cookies and milky products from cows will be enough to do it. It is possible that you have less swollen hemorrhoids which remain inside the rectum, so that you may not always see them. They can be sore, itchy, even bleed at times.

MY 10-POINT HEMORRHOID ACTION PLAN

1 Try a rotation of the following natural herbal creams. You can buy them in a health food store. Start with the first cream and continue use until the hemorrhoids disappear, or the cream runs out. If the cream runs out, and you still have the hemorrhoids, then start on the second herbal cream and so on.
(a) *Hamamelis Virginica* (witch hazel), especially if the hemorrhoids are painful to touch. Witch hazel compresses can help to constrict and shrink the veins.
(b) *Pilewort* ointment
(c) *Horse chestnut* ointment
(d) *Plantain and Yarrow* ointment

2 Try the following homeopathic remedies:
(a) *Hamamelis* 30 c – if the hemorrhoids are painful to touch, bruised, sore
(b) *Sulfur* 30 c – if hemorrhoids are hot, on fire, burning and/or itching
(c) *Sepia* 30 c – if hemorrhoids feel like a ball on your rectum.

3 Drink extra dandelion tea to clear congestion of the liver (3 or 4 cups a day).

4 Sit in a basin of cold water. This may sound shocking, but it will help lessen inflammation and reduce the engorged blood vessels.

5 Apply green clay (available from a health food store). Mix it with water. It's messy, but may relieve the swelling and pain. To remove the clay, take a bath or shower.

6 Add the herb bilberry to your dietary regimen. It is high in bioflavonoids, which are anti-inflammatory compounds that help to relieve hemorrhoids. Take 1 capsule of bilberry every hour in acute cases until healed.

7 Add 1 tablespoon of flax oil to your diet and take before each meal.

8 Take 1 capsule of milk thistle twice a day to help soften the stool and cleanse the liver.

9 Don't strain on the toilet. This will only make matters worse.

10 Eat liver-building foods such as cabbage, broccoli and Brussels sprouts. Learn to sprout your own broccoli seeds (see page 213).

SIGNS OF A TIRED BLADDER

Is this you?

► Poor bladder control
► Scanty/dark/cloudy urine
► Urinating every five minutes
► Stiffness in your little toe
► Headaches

URINE

DIFFICULTY IN PEEING

If you feel the need to pee, but it won't come out easily, this is a sign that you need to balance your bladder and kidney energies. You can do that with the foods and herbs listed in the bladder chart below.

Solutions:

► Eat the foods and herbs listed in the bladder chart on page 51. If the problem persists, see a specialist.
► Try eating quinoa (see page 212). It's one of the best kidney/bladder foods.

TOO MUCH PEE AND ALWAYS RUNNING TO THE LOO

I am talking about every fifteen to thirty minutes. This is a sign of low kidney energy and a tired bladder. It can also be caused by drinking too many soft drinks loaded with sugar and additives.

Solutions:

► Introduce barley, wheat berries, sweet rice, aduki beans, black beans, kidney beans, wild salmon and trout into your diet to help your kidneys. Also add parsley to savory foods where possible.
► If you are prone to bladder infections, try eating cranberries or drinking cranberry juice (cranberries are the best fruit for the bladder); make soups or broths from veggies that are effective for the bladder, such as celery, carrots, squash, asparagus and lima beans; drink dandelion tea and eat flax seeds.

McKEITH BLADDER BUILDER PROGRAM

Be sure to include plenty of the following in your daily diet:

▸ **BEANS**
Aduki
Kidney
Lima

▸ **SEA VEGETABLES**
Kombu
Wakame
Nori

▸ **FISH**
Trout
Wild salmon

▸ **FLUIDS**
Cranberry/cherry juice
Nettle/dandelion tea
Plenty of water
Soups made from celery, carrots,
squash, asparagus, lima beans

▸ **HERBS**
The herb Uva Ursi
(500mg twice a day)
works wonders.

▸ **AVOID**
Caffeine
Coffee
Tea (with caffeine)

CLOUDY URINE

A sign that your body is damp and acidic, due to eating the wrong foods. Sugars, animal products, dairy, eggs and refined grains such as white rice and too much wheat acidify your insides, producing large amounts of chlorine and toxins. When the body is overly acidic it becomes a breeding ground for bacteria. Some people with cloudy urine exhibit other symptoms of damp such as lethargy, heavy limbs, sluggishness, a feeling of stiffness and a fuzzy head.

Solutions:

▸ Eat the superfood wild blue-green algae to help dry up the damp.

▸ Also aduki beans, millet, turnips, sweet potatoes and other root vegetables.

GET TO KNOW YOUR BODY

PIMPLES

Pimples point to congestion or imbalances. Depending on where they are situated on the body, you can tell which organ is affected.

PIMPLES ON: BODY PART AFFECTED

FOREHEAD: INTESTINAL AREA
Solutions:
- Clean yourself out with 1 tablespoon of psyllium husks daily in water.
- Give yourself regular enemas or even get a few colonics. (See page 151.)

CHEEKS: LUNGS AND BREAST AREA
Solutions:
- Drink mullein tea and take astragalus supplements, three times a day.
- Take oil of evening primrose supplements (1000mg daily).
- Take echinacea liquid tincture (20 drops twice a day).
- Avoid cow's milk products, saturated fats and red meats.

NOSE: HEART AREA
Solutions:
- Take hawthorn supplements, 500mg twice daily plus 100mg coenzyme Q10.
- Eat barley grass (1 teaspoon a day).
- Drink 2 cups of hawthorn tea daily.

JAW: KIDNEY AREA
Solutions:
- Eat quinoa.
- Drink dandelion teas.
- Take a magnesium supplement (1000mcg daily) and B complex (100mg daily).

SHOULDER: DIGESTIVE AREA
Solutions:
- Take digestive enzyme supplements with all meals.
- Drink 1 tablespoon of aloe vera juice before meals.

CHEST: LUNG AND HEART AREA
Solutions:
- Drink mullein teas and ginkgo biloba teas regularly.
- Take coenzyme Q10 supplements (100mg daily).
- Sprinkle lecithin granules on salads and cereals.

UPPER BACK: LUNG AREA
Solutions:
- Take astragalus (500mg twice a day)
- Take germanium supplements (200mg daily).
- Include the following herbs in your food preparation: basil, cayenne, fennel, fenugreek, garlic, ginger, mullein, nettles, peppermint.
- Drink celery juice and mullein teas.
- Eat simple, small meals avoiding dairy products and sugars.
- Cut out peanuts for a while.

AROUND THE MOUTH: REPRODUCTIVE AREA
Solution:
- The herb agnus castus can help to correct hormonal imbalances that manifest as pimples around the mouth. Take this supplement twice a day.

EXCESSIVE YAWNING AND SIGHING

It is not always a sign that you are bored. You are probably running on empty and may be suffering from hypoglycemia (low blood sugar).

Solutions:

- ► Take a teaspoon of the superfood spirulina twice a day, morning and afternoon. Or try my Living Food Energy Powder to balance your blood (available in health food stores).
- ► Fifteen drops of ginseng tincture in a tiny amount of water *after meals* could help regulate your blood sugar.

My goal in helping you get to know your body is to show just how much of an effect food has on your body and how you feel each day. These basic tips could make an amazing difference, and you will also likely find that you start listening to your body beyond the signs listed in this chapter. You'll soon detect whether a food makes you feel vital and healthy, or gives you a bloated stomach or a headache! This knowledge is powerful – it's the key to really living and experiencing health at the highest level.

CHAPTER 3

THE DIET OF ABUNDANCE: EAT MORE NOT LESS

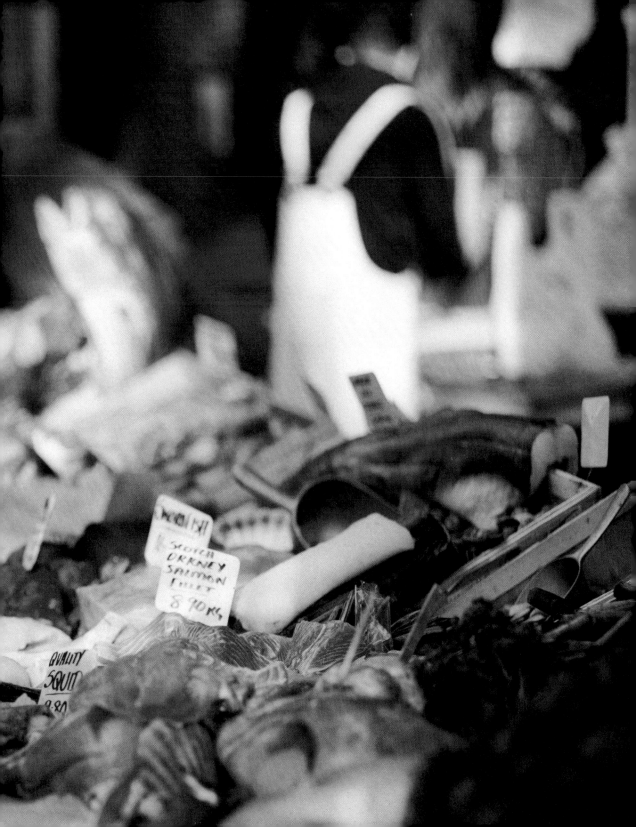

EVEN A MINOR SHIFT IN YOUR EATING HABITS CAN TRANSFORM YOUR WHOLE SENSE OF WELL-BEING. MY EMPHASIS IS NOT ABOUT TELLING YOU WHAT NOT TO EAT BUT IN TURNING YOU ON TO HUNDREDS OF NEW FOODS THAT YOU MAY NEVER HAVE KNOWN ABOUT. THIS ISN'T A DIET OF RESTRICTION – RATHER, IT'S ONE OF ABUNDANCE. I WANT YOU TO EAT MORE FOODS, NOT LESS. I WANT TO SHATTER YOUR EXPECTATIONS OF DIETING.

IN MY OWN CLINICAL PRACTICE, PATIENTS WHO FIRST COME TO ME WANTING TO LOSE WEIGHT (HOWEVER MUCH), END UP ACHIEVING THEIR DESIRED GOAL AND LOOKING FANTASTIC. BUT THEY NEED TO MAKE THE COMMITMENT TO EATING MORE OF MY HEALTHY FOODS, AND LESS OF THE UNHEALTHY FOODS. AND I PROMISE THAT IF YOU FOLLOW MY DIET OF ABUNDANCE, YOU WILL NEVER HAVE A WEIGHT PROBLEM.

NICHOLAS MADE THAT COMMITMENT, BUT JUST LOOK AT HOW HIS FOOD DIARY SHAPED UP BEFORE COMING ON *YOU ARE WHAT YOU EAT* ...

NICHOLAS'S FOOD DIARY

MONDAY

2am 3 slices of deep pan pizza

10am Coffee – strong with semi-skimmed milk

1pm Coffee

3pm Coffee

4pm Coffee

5pm Coffee

8pm ½ bottle vodka with 1 liter orange juice

10pm 4 small onion bhajis, 6 small mushroom bhajis
½ deep pan spicy chicken pizza

11pm ½ pint caramel ice cream

During night 4 pints of water

TUESDAY

7am Coffee

10am 6 beef sandwiches: 12 slices small white bread,
6 slices beef from local deli (380g), spreadable light butter
2 cans fizzy orange

12pm Tea with milk and 2 sugars

2pm Coffee

4pm Chicken sandwich (prepackaged): brown bread, mayo and salad

7pm 5 pints of beer, 4 bottles of lager (9 ounces)

10:30pm 3 slices of deep pan ham and pineapple pizza

WEDNESDAY

8am–12pm 4 coffees

2 pieces of haddock in breadcrumbs
(frozen prepackaged) with 2 tablespoons butter

4pm Cheese and onion quiche

9pm Store-bought fish and chips with brown sauce

THURSDAY

2am 2 cheese sandwiches: 4 slices medium white bread with
butter, 4^1/$_2$oz red cheese, small onion

7am Coffee

9am Coffee

5–7pm 1^1/$_2$ liters sherry

9pm ^{1}/$_2$lb burger with large portion of oven French fries, 2 fried eggs
(in lard), tomato ketchup, 3 slices white bread, butter

11pm Tea with milk and 2 sugars

FRIDAY

5am 3 cheese sandwiches: 6 large slices white bread with
butter, 5oz red cheese, small onion

8am Coffee

12pm Can of meatballs in onion gravy, large portion of oven
fries, 2 large prepackaged luxury pork sausages, 4 large
slices white bread, butter

2pm 3 beef sandwiches: 6 large slices white bread, butter,
4oz prepackaged sliced beef

3pm Tea with milk and 2 sugars

5pm Coffee

10pm 4 bags of potato chips, 18oz chocolates,
6 chocolate-coated after-dinner mints

SATURDAY

1am ½ homemade lasagne: 1lb lean minced steak fried in olive oil, 2 tins of mushrooms, 2 onions, 2 jars of tomato sauce, 6 strips dried lasagne

2am Can of fizzy orange

8am ½ homemade lasagne

8am Coffee

10am Coffee, 10oz chocolates, 6 chocolate-coated after-dinner mints, 2oz bar dairy milk chocolate with caramel

12pm Coffee

2pm Tea with milk and 2 sugars

3pm 2lbs stewing steak, 2 packages of beef casserole mix

6pm Can of rice pudding

10pm Whole 11-inch deep pan spicy chicken pizza, 6 small mushroom bhajis, tea with milk and 2 sugars

SUNDAY

3am Mince and onion (big plateful left over from Saturday) ⅕lb mashed potatoes

9am 4 slices of bacon, 2 eggs fried in butter, 14oz can of sausages and beans, 2 coffees

1pm 1 pint tub of caramel ice cream

4pm 2½lb roasted chicken, 6 mashed potatoes with cream and butter, can processed peas, 6 medium carrots

5pm Can of rice pudding

6pm Coffee

8pm Mug of hot malted milk with 1 sugar and 2 marshmallows

SO YOU THINK YOU HAVE A HEALTHY DIET?

The first big issue I run into at the clinic is when I ask the new patient about the quality of his/her diet. Inevitably, most patients tell me they eat a healthy diet. It is only after probing, questioning and asking them to provide a detailed food inventory for the week that we discover that most people eat terribly, even when they think they're eating just fine. So, before we go much further, I would like you to complete my Food Intelligence Quotient Test (FIT-IQ) now.

Depending on your FIT-IQ grade, you will either be able to quickly skim this chapter, using it as a simple reference guide (if you're a high FIT-IQer), or, alternatively, will have to keep this chapter – and this book – with you at all times, and never let it out of your sight!

DR. GILLIAN'S FOOD INTELLIGENCE (QUOTIENT) TEST

Answer Yes or No to the following questions:

1 Do you eat at least one piece of raw fruit each day?

2 Do you eat at least five servings of vegetables each day?

3 Do you eat rice, quinoa, millet, oats or other grains at least three times a week?

4 Do you eat a serving of raw vegetables each day?

5 Do you eat raw seeds at least three times a week?

6 Do you use seaweed in your cooking?

7 Do you include fish in your diet at least twice a week?

8 Do you chew your food thoroughly until it's liquefied?

9 Do you go out of your way to avoid foods containing preservatives, additives, colorings or E numbers?

10 Do you avoid foods that contain sugar or added sugar?

11 If you are stressed do you wait until the feeling has passed before eating?

12 Were you breast-fed as a child?

13 Do you always make sure that you take time to eat properly, even if you feel tired or busy?

14 Do you eat breakfast every day?

15 Do you drink bottled spring water every day?

16 Do you drink at least eight glasses of filtered, spring or mineral water every day?

17 Do you avoid beer/alcohol/ soda when eating?

18 Do you drink water approximately 25 minutes before eating your main meals, instead of drinking water with meals?

19 Do you eat a varied diet instead of eating the same foods every day?

20 Do you make raw vegetable juices at least once a week?

YOUR SCORE

Add up the number of your Yes answers.

17–20: EXCELLENT – TOP OF THE CLASS
Please look at this chapter, familiarize yourself with it, and you should be just fine.

12–16: NOT BAD – COULD TRY HARDER
You're trying, which is good news, but not hard enough. You had better study this chapter – and this book – faithfully! I expect you to make a real effort to do most of what I am telling you. Start following my Diet of Abundance at your earliest convenience.

11 OR LESS: YOU'RE FLUNKING OUT!
STOP! Don't move! I am really worried about you. You are in a serious mess. I am ordering you to take to heart every word of this chapter and book. I am literally *begging* you to start my Diet of Abundance today, without delay.

Let's start with some very simple quick preliminary eating tips:

▶ Go for variety in your diet. It will deliver more nutrients and make you feel more satisfied.
▶ Add one or two new foods each week to your routine diet.
▶ Eat organically grown foods where available.
▶ Use whole grains instead of refined processed grains and brown rice instead of white. Whole grain flour, bread and spaghetti are better than refined flour.
▶ Take a break from wheat whenever possible and introduce other grains such as barley, spelt, millet, amaranth, quinoa and rye.
▶ Eat fresh vegetables every day.
▶ Use unrefined sea salt instead of regular table salt.
▶ Use unrefined cold-pressed oils, such as sesame, corn, olive, sunflower.
▶ Use no-added-sugar jams.
▶ Drink pure (not concentrated) fruit juices.
▶ Rice syrup and barley syrup are better natural sweeteners than white sugar.
▶ Eat white wild fish (not farmed) rather than meat and chicken.
▶ Eat protein foods such as beans, tofu, quinoa and tempeh instead of meat and cheese.
▶ Use sea vegetables for your cooking (see page 207). These vegetables are a valuable source of nutrients, including calcium, beta-carotene and vitamin B12, which help reduce cholesterol, rid the body of toxins and strengthen immunity.
▶ Introduce new foods into your life and eat more of them, especially from my List of Abundance (page 82). Be open-minded!

How fantastic is it that you don't need to feel hungry again? At the beginning of their transformation, the biggest concern of the participants on my TV show was "Will I be hungry?"

On my Diet of Abundance, you will end up eating a much wider variety of foods than you ever thought possible. And the beauty of it is that you can eat as much of these foods as you like. Your cravings will be banished for good because you will finally be feeding your body.

MAKING THE CHANGE

Joanne, a participant on my TV show who had lived her entire life on burgers and a very limited diet, was extremely worried about how hard it would be to change. She thought I could not possibly understand what she was going through. How wrong could she be.

Many years ago, when I moved away from home to go to university, I survived on a very stodgy diet of saturated meat and potatoes, drank dozens of cups of caffeinated tea until buzzing point and snacked on bags of potato chips. I then moved to Spain for a year, and lived on a regimen of chocolate éclairs and Spanish pastries with a few sangrias to wash them down, as well as processed white rice and pork chops. I was overweight and totally depleted of nutrients. Needless to say, I had no energy, my skin was a big mess and I felt quite sick.

I dragged myself kicking and screaming to change my ways. It was not easy and took a while. But the transformation in my health was worth the effort. The participants on the show were forced to make their changes in only eight weeks! I want you to take the time you need to make these changes, but the good news is that you will start to feel the benefits almost immediately.

Once you have reached your health goal, I often tell my patients if you follow the 80/20 rule, you will be fine. Do what I suggest 80 percent of the time and that leaves a 20 percent window of food naughtiness. But you might just find that your body does not want to be food naughty. It likes the new you and does not want to spoil the exhilarating feeling. If you do indeed cheat, don't beat yourself up. Accept it, then get back on track.

So challenge yourself and open your mind to the new possibilities. I bet you have no idea how well you can really feel, how much energy you can attain, how sharp your mind could really be, how much happiness you can exude, until you take the steps. It's almost like if you never get your eyes tested, you have no idea how well you can see. If you don't challenge yourself with your health and offer your body good food, you have no idea just how great you can feel.

If you eat dead, lifeless food, your body will be lifeless. If you eat vital, vibrant foods with lots of fresh fruits and veggies, you will be full of life force and vitality too. It's the way it works. It's that simple.

In Nepal, amaranth seeds are eaten as porridge called "sattoo" or milled into flour to make chapatis. Amaranth can be cooked as a cereal, ground into flour, popped like popcorn, sprouted or toasted. The seeds can be cooked with other whole grains, added to stir-fries or to soups and stews as a nutrient-dense thickening agent.

ENERGY GRAINS

Rich in nutrients, grains are your basic energy food. Almost all whole, unrefined grains can be beneficial to your health, while refined grains, such as white rice, white bread and white pasta, are devoid of most nutrients and fiber due to the refining process. These processed grains behave like sugar when eaten, rushing into the blood system and causing havoc. This can result in blood sugar imbalances, sugar cravings, mood swings and weight gain. That's why a healthy diet should always include the unrefined versions of grains such as brown rice, pot barley, amaranth, millet, rye groats, wheat berries, buckwheat groats and so on. Generally, the darker the color, the more unrefined the grain and the healthier it is for you. Here are some of the grains I recommend.

AMARANTH
Amaranth is very strengthening to the lungs – so very beneficial in these days of high pollution and ozone intoxication. And it contains even more calcium and magnesium than cow's milk!

BARLEY
Two types of barley are available: pearl barley is the refined version; pot barley is the whole grain. Go for the pot barley. Barley is sweet tasting and good for your stomach and digestion. If you suffer from indigestion, barley can make a difference. It does have some gluten but levels are low. (Note: Barley is not to be confused with the superfood barley grass. Barley grass does not contain gluten.)

BROWN RICE
Brown rice is extremely beneficial for the nervous and digestive systems. Of all the grains, it is the least allergenic – even for the most sensitive individuals.
Rice Rules
▶ Short grain: Eat in autumn and winter to warm your insides.
▶ Long grain: Eat in summer to keep you cool.
▶ Basmati: Perfect for people who are overweight or internally damp with mucus and catarrh.

BUCKWHEAT GROATS
Buckwheat groats are gluten-free, rich in healthy minerals and (unlike wheat) are nonallergenic. If you are sensitive to wheat, this is a superb alternative for you. It contains a decent amount of protein, about 20 percent, as well as the bioflavanoid rutin, which helps strengthen circulation and veins. If you suffer from varicose veins, this is the grain for you. Great for livening up salads.

CORN

Also known as maize, corn is very common. You will find it in a lot of baked goods. When ground, corn is often added to prepackaged foods. As a result, corn is a bit like wheat: added to too many foods and, as a result, a potential allergenic if you eat too much of it. To release the nutrients from corn kernels, you need to chew the kernels really well as the skin is indigestible.

KAMUT

Kamut is closely related to wheat, but many wheat-sensitive people tolerate kamut. It contains twice as much protein as wheat, more minerals, especially magnesium and zinc, as well as sixteen amino acids and essential fatty acids too.

MILLET

Millet is an excellent grain food source. High in iron, magnesium, potassium, the B vitamins and vitamin E, it supports the digestive system, improves nutrient uptake and is a great energy booster as it supports the spleen, your energy battery.

QUINOA

Quinoa (pronounced *keenwa*) is a South American grain that is becoming more widely available and contains all the essential amino acids. It is therefore a complete protein but is more easier to digest than meat protein and has a far lower fat content than most meat.

OATS

Oats contain more good fats than other grains – fats that will help you to actually lose weight, not gain it. Oats are also a rich source of vitamin B complex, good for the nervous system and for strengthening your bones.

RYE

A good grain for sourdough baking. Some of my patients grow sprouts from the rye berries (see page 213 for growing sprouts). Rye is excellent for the liver. Make a broth with the grain if you are a headache sufferer.

SPELT

Spelt, like buckwheat groats, is loaded with minerals and protein, and strengthening to the constitutional organs. It is a tasty, nourishing alternative for those sensitive to wheat. Constipation, colitis and poor digestion are some of the conditions spelt can help. It's the only grain that contains mucopolysaccharides which stimulate the immune system. It's a good source of constant energy.

TEFF

Teff is a tiny seed with lots of flavor. Its high protein content provides good levels of calcium, magnesium and iron, making it a good choice for people who are salt cravers. Teff contains more potassium than most other grains, helping to clear poor diet acids from the blood.

WHAT ABOUT WHEAT?

Most of us eat far too much wheat. Although it's a healthy grain, eating too much of it can ultimately exert a negative effect on the blood and organs, leading to food intolerances and allergies. It has, in fact, become highly allergenic due to its excessive intake in the West. I recommend you substitute other grains for wheat wherever possible, but don't worry about eating whole wheat in moderation.

HELPFUL HINTS ABOUT GRAINS

▶ Eat only unrefined grains, not processed ones.

▶ Wash grains well before cooking.

▶ Cook until the grains are soft and all the water has been absorbed (see Grain Cooking Chart, this page).

▶ Chew grains well. This will improve digestion.

▶ Did you know the gluten content of wheat virtually disappears, once germinated via sprouts? Try sprouting your favorite grains (see page 213 for sprouting instructions).

▶ Store grains in sealed containers, and use within four months of purchasing. A bay leaf can be added to keep cereal-nibbling critters away. I normally keep my own grains in the fridge or freezer (especially during warm summer months).

COOKING WITH GRAINS

GRAIN	AMOUNT OF GRAIN IN CUPS	AMOUNT OF WATER IN CUPS	COOKING TIME IN MINUTES
▶ Amaranth	1	2½	35
▶ Brown rice	1	2	20–35
▶ Buckwheat (roasted)	1	2	20
▶ Millet	1	3	30–45
▶ Oats (whole groats)	1	2	45–60
▶ Pot barley	1	3	45–60
▶ Quinoa	1	2	8–12

Note: If you soak the grains for a few hours prior to use, you may be able to reduce your cooking time by half.

BOUNTIFUL BEANS

Also known as legumes or pulses, beans are basically seeds from a pod of a specific group of plants. Most of them are packed with complete protein and contain almost no fat.

Beans are great for weight loss. They also lower cholesterol, prevent heart disease and purge the body of unwanted toxins. Finally, they are a good source of complex carbohydrates, the good healthy type. Because the truth is that carbohydrates such as beans, grains and veggies are essential to our biochemistry and physiology. We need them to be healthy, strong, and even to flourish as a species. If you don't eat enough good carbohydrates you will feel ill.

All my patients who stopped eating carbohydrates became weak, constipated, gaunt, irritable and depressed. It's like playing Russian roulette with your body. I agree th. it's a good idea to cut out the bad refined carbohydrates such as cakes, cookies, biscuits and sweets. But the message here needs to be very clear: Complex carbohydrates, such as beans, are essential for good health! Eat them regularly.

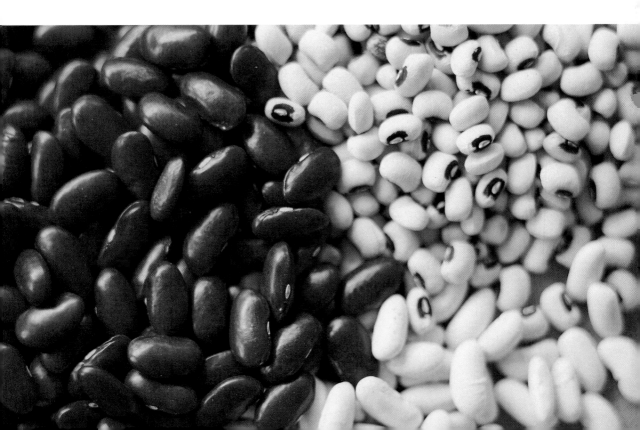

ADUKI: THE WEIGHT LOSS BEAN

Aduki beans are an excellent bean food source, high in nutrients but low in calories. In Japan, aduki beans are noted for their healing qualities, and are used in the treatment of kidney and bladder infections. But in my own clinical practice, I use them for patients who need to lose weight. This bean, with its exceptionally high levels of fiber, vitamin B complex and minerals (iron, manganese and zinc), acts as a natural diuretic to relieve the body of excess fluids. It also removes unwanted mucus, congestion and stools, burns fat and balances metabolism for weight management. If you want to lose weight, this is the bean for you.

MUNG: THE DETOX BEAN

Mung beans are another good food source. I have used this bean in my practice to help lower high blood pressure, treat gastrointestinal ulcers and urinary problems, and to cleanse the blood by introducing more oxygen. They are a wonderful liver cleanser and I have always incorporated mung beans in my detox at the clinic.

FAVA, SOY AND LENTILS: THE MEAT BEANS

Fava, soy and lentils are all high protein, and gram for gram they are even more efficient complete protein providers than red meat – without the fat content. In addition to their perfect protein profile, lentils also nourish the kidneys and adrenal glands, while fava beans are high in amino acids, B vitamins, calcium and iron. Soybeans have become a popular alternative to meat due to their complete protein content. They also contain several anti-cancer compounds including phytoestrogen, and have a balancing effect on both male and female hormones.

Every cell in your body needs protein; it is required for the growth and repair of everything from muscles and bones to hair and fingernails. Protein also helps us create enzymes that enable us to digest food, produce antibodies that fight off infection and hormones that keep the body working efficiently.

GO WILD

I prefer wild fish from the seas instead of farmed fish, since the farms tend to be overcrowded, thus sometimes breeding illness. Go for fish from less polluted waters.

SOURCES OF PROTEIN

Although protein is vital for our health and well-being, eating too much isn't good for you as the body cannot store the protein it doesn't immediately need. Instead, the liver converts excess protein into glucose and toxins, which increases your risk of poor health and weight gain.

Meat, fish, poultry, eggs and milk are rich sources of protein but they aren't the best sources as the liver finds it hard to digest all that fat as well as the antibiotics and other chemicals used in the raising of animal produce. Your body simply has to work a lot harder to digest meat proteins.

It's far better to vary your protein sources and get some protein from less well-known sources, such as grains. Many grains are superb sources of protein, in particular quinoa, which is a more usable protein than meat, but also buckwheat, millet and amaranth, legumes, nuts, seeds, green leafy vegetables and sprouted seeds.

All soybean products, such as tofu and soymilk, are good sources. If you do eat meat, avoid red meat and go for lean meats, such as turkey and chicken, which have a lower fat content, and oily fish which is rich in essential fatty acids. When choosing dairy products, opt for the low-fat variety so you get the protein but not the fat.

FISH

Choose from non-fatty white meat fish, such as carp, cod, haddock, trout or, occasionally, organic or wild salmon. Oily fish are rich in essential fatty acids, and very good for regulating hormone and blood sugar levels when considering weight management.

NUTS AND SEEDS

Nuts and seeds should be included in your diet regularly. These contain high levels of essential fatty acids (EFAs), or good fats. When you eat these good fats you won't put on weight – they even help you lose excess weight.

Nuts and seeds contain a powerhouse of other nutrients, especially the full profile of amino acids needed to form complete and digestible protein, plus vitamins A, B, C and E and the minerals calcium, magnesium, potassium, zinc, iron, potassium, selenium and manganese. Sunflower seeds, flax seeds (or linseeds), alfalfa seeds, pumpkin seeds, sesame seeds, almonds, chestnuts, cashews, pecans, brazil nuts and walnuts are particularly beneficial.

Nuts and seeds are so nutrient-dense that you don't need to eat a lot of them – a teaspoon or two a day, or every other day, would more than do. Use them in cooking as garnishes or to flavor a gourmet dish, sprinkle them on your breakfast cereal or simply eat them as an ideal snack by itself. I often soak my raw nuts or seeds in water for several hours. It gives them a lovely texture and consistency and makes them easier to digest. Try soaking your almonds – you'll love it. For a fluffy topping for desserts and puddings, try soaking raw cashews for a few hours, then put them in a blender and whip up into a cream.

GOOD SWEETS

Not all sweets are bad for you. In fact, almost all the sweets given to us by Mother Nature are great for us. These are, literally, the fruits of the Earth. Fruits are nutrient-rich and a great source of live enzymes and antioxidants to boost your immune system and energy levels. The best fruits include blueberries, blackberries, raspberries, strawberries, watermelon, apples, apricots, cherries, grapes, peaches, pears, plums, raisins and tangerines. I recommend you eat at least one or two fresh raw seasonal fruits every day.

Sweeteners that are fine to use occasionally as snacks or in cooking are brown rice syrup, rice and barley malt, honey, molasses, diluted apple juice, diluted grape juice and pure maple syrup.

I won't let you get sugared out . . .

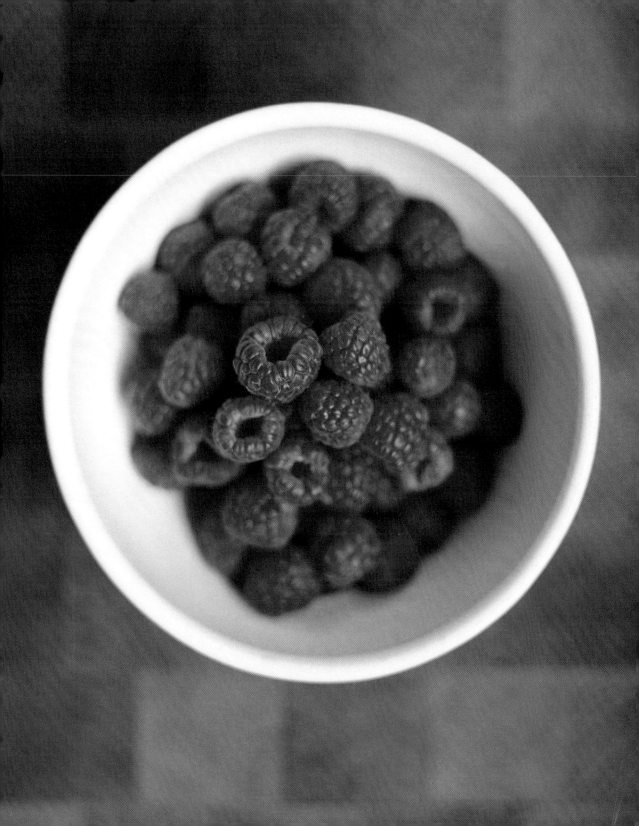

THE NASTIES CHALLENGE

I make my own patients fill out food and drink inventories for at least ten days before they come to see me. They have to write the time and details of everything they eat and drink for that ten-day period. They also keep a track of moods, feelings and health complaints alongside the foods for each day. This data can provide a fantastic insight into a person's life. Often I will tell people to bring in the wrappers of prepackaged foods and canned foods they have eaten so that we can go through ingredients they may have eaten without realizing.

The Nasties Challenge is designed to make you think about any bad habits you have and what it means to your health. So, put your hand on heart and be completely honest here.

How many of the following do you consume on average in a week? Keep a tally of your scores.

- Cups of coffee

- Cups of regular tea

- Fried food

- Frozen dinners/fast/packaged foods

- Chocolate

- Sweets

- Pasta

- Baked goods

- Sugar in your tea or coffee

- Canned food with added salt

- Red meat

- Non-organic poultry

- Glasses of cow's milk

- Slices of white bread

- Units of alcohol (on average a small glass of wine is 1 unit and a pint of lager is 2)

BELOW 15: GREAT! YOU MAY BE ELIGIBLE AS A "DR. GILLIAN GROUPIE"!

You should be proud. Please keep up the good work. Your long-term prospects for a healthy life are superb.

SCORE: 15–25: GETTING THERE

You are the kind of person who could easily cut out the rubbish in your diet. It's not too late. Maybe you are bored? Life is a bit dull. Get some exercise, take up a hobby. You do not feel quite as good as you could and you know it. Do something about it now.

SCORE: 26–50: YOU ARE A PLAYER

You are dumbing yourself down and playing with your health. But ask yourself: for what reason? Do you need to get ill before you make the change? What's it going to take? Follow my Detox Day (see page 140) this weekend and get back on track. Make a promise to yourself to do better. You are worth it.

SCORE 51–100: YOU ARE A BIG MESS. YOU'RE NOT OKAY!

I am *not* happy, and you shouldn't be either, because you are a mess waiting to happen. You are playing Russian roulette with your health and body, and I'm worried. Even if you think that everything is fine right now, your lifestyle and diet will eventually catch up with you. So your long-term prospects are downright scary, if you don't do what I am telling you.

SCORE 101–150: YOU FLUNK, BIG TIME!

This is really bad. You should be ashamed of yourself! Either shape up by reducing your score with my advice in this book, or you're wasting my time. I am begging you, *ordering* you, to make significant changes, starting today. Time is a matter of urgency in your case.

NOTE TO SMOKERS

Smoking strips your body of vital nutrients, prevents nutrient uptake from food, weakens your digestion and poisons your blood.

THE DIET OF ABUNDANCE

THE NASTIES

There are certain foods – the nasties – that must be avoided. You must either delete these cold-turkey, or at the very least, cut down on them significantly. The bad nasties can be downright harmful and counterproductive in getting you the results that you want. I don't want to get hung up on telling you what not to eat or do. My emphasis is exploring the exciting new food choices and fun new lifestyle that we can embark upon together. I've given you a short list of bad nasties below, to keep things simple. You'll see that there aren't that many of them, and I hope this will encourage you more. But please, I repeat *please*, accommodate my requests here. Ultimately you will be delighted, thankful and looking and feeling like a million bucks!

Here's my short list of Bad Nasties.

COFFEE

Coffee contains caffeine – a stimulant drug also present in tea and cola drinks. When you drink too much coffee, your blood pressure rises, leaving you feeling anxious and restless. The paradox is that although coffee is a stimulant, it overworks the adrenal glands, tiring out both them and you.

Moreover, all coffee, even decaf, can stimulate skin aging. It also reduces the absorption of iron and zinc by up to 50 percent, which can compromise your immune system. Wean yourself off coffee slowly. Instead, start drinking a rotation of herbal teas, such as peppermint, camomile, dandelion, nettle and red clover, or simply some freshly squeezed fruit juice in hot water.

FATTY FOODS

Too many fatty foods, including red meats, dairy products, fried and "junk" foods, can clog the arteries, deplete calcium levels and compromise the function of the heart and other vital organs. There's no diplomatic way to put this, but excessive intake of fatty foods makes you fat. It also leads to high blood pressure, food allergies, heart disease, diabetes, eating disorders, liver and kidney problems, osteoporosis, arthritis, colon, breast and uterine cancers.

SWEET FOODS

Too many sweet foods and refined white sugar, dextrose, corn syrup, artificial sweeteners and chocolate can cause severe blood sugar imbalances, mood swings, a lower resistance to infection, hyperactivity and hamper the function of the spleen, liver, pancreas and intestines. Use alternative natural sweeteners such as honey, molasses and pure fruits and juices, but use them sparingly.

DAIRY PRODUCTS

Cow's milk is high in fat and the protein casein, which is hard for humans to digest properly. This is why cow's milk can trigger allergic responses such as asthma, earache, runny nose, catarrh, skin rash, lethargy and irritability.

Furthermore, some people lack the enzyme lactase, which breaks down lactose in milk. If you are lactose intolerant you may suffer from bloating, wind, flatulence, diarrhea or constipation. Instead, try the more easily digestible alternative goat's milk or soy, rice, nut, triple grain and oat milks. If you cut out dairy foods, keep your calcium intake up by eating calcium-rich foods such as tofu, legumes, nuts and seeds and leafy greens; amaranth (see page 64) is also very high in calcium and magnesium.

Finally, if you really must drink cow's milk, then please boil it first. The boiling process breaks down the large indigestible molecules.

ALCOHOL

Alcohol puts a big strain on your digestive system and liver. The liver converts alcohol into acetaldehyde, a toxic cousin of formaldehyde used in tanning leather and the embalming process. Too much alcohol can lead to obesity and its connected problems, blood sugar imbalances, fatigue, sluggish organs and cell tissue degeneration.

Too much coffee can make you susceptible to colds and flu.

THE SO-SO FOODS: PROCEED WITH CAUTION

You don't need to avoid these foods forever, but just know to eat them only in moderation. In other words, proceed with a bit of caution here.

YEASTS

Nearly all baked goods contain added yeast as a raising agent and to enhance flavor. If your baked good is raised or has a crust, it will undoubtedly contain yeast. Packaged goods often contain yeast additives which might be described as autolyzed yeast protein, yeast extract, hydrolyzed vegetable protein, vegetable protein, baker's yeast, brewer's and torula yeast, so read the label before buying. Fermented foods (e.g., vinegar, soy sauce, cheese) and alcoholic beverages (especially wine and beer) are another source of yeast. Yeasts are problems only to those who are sensitive to them: if you suffer from allergies, candidiasis, asthma, yeast infections, eczema, hives, headaches or migraines, then the chances are you will need to eliminate excess yeast.

Yeast sensitivities can be created by eating too many of these "yeasties," as I call them. I'm not saying that you must never eat foods with yeast. I just want you to be aware that you should limit your intake of yeast-containing foods. A final note: Most baked goods are made with loads of added sugars too. So, occasional treat, not a dietary staple.

PASTA

If you think white pasta is a nutrient-dense food, think again. Commercial pasta is made from white flour. Refining and bleaching destroys at least 70 percent of its vitamin content and up to 90 percent of its mineral content. White flour is devoid of fiber, very low in minerals and contains *inorganic* iron, which can accumulate in the body (*inorganic* iron depletes other good vitamins). I'm not saying you can *never* eat white pasta; but I am asking you to eat it in moderation.

My best advice here is to introduce other types of pastas into your diet. Instead of white pasta, better choices could be rice, spinach, spelt, corn and soy pastas, all of which are available in health food stores and even some supermarkets.

RED MEAT

Too much red meat can toxify and acidify the blood, deplete calcium, overwork the kidneys and liver and stagnate in the intestines, killing the beneficial flora. This can lead to kidney stones, a sluggish liver and/or liver disease, bowel and reproductive cancers, arthritis and osteoporosis. Red meat puts a strain on the body's ability to produce enzymes and hydrochloric acid, which are necessary for digestion. If you are eating red meat, learn to food combine properly so that you make your digestion of the meat more effective (see page 78). And try to eat organic meats wherever possible.

NIGHTSHADES

Avoid foods from the nightshade family of foods (tomatoes, potatoes, aubergines and peppers) if you are prone to muscular, arthritic, joint or bone problems.

Arthritic sufferers need to especially avoid the nightshades because they contain a substance called solanine, which interferes with the enzymes in the muscles, often causing pain and discomfort and aggravating joint problems. If you really love these foods, the best thing you can do is to roast, bake or cook these veggies with a little miso soup. This process will neutralize the solanine compound.

POULTRY

The process by which commercial chickens are reared means that diseased animals may land on your plate. Therefore, I recommend that you eat organic poultry if available.

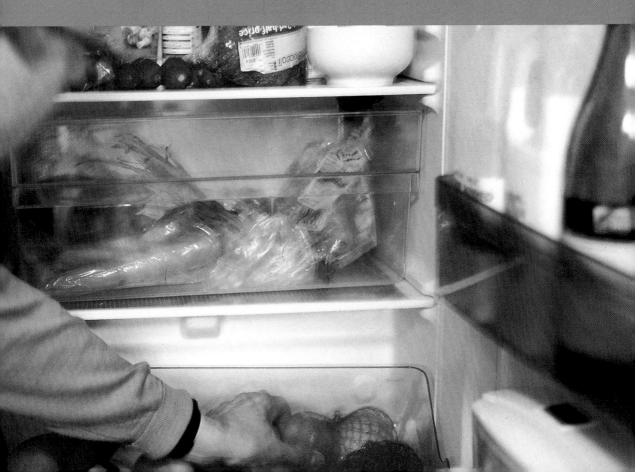

FOOD COMBINING

Many of my patients come to me for help with their diets. Most of these people have been overweight, gassy and bloated after meals. Food combining can provide the perfect solution. When you food combine, fat is able to burn away properly; so you are not left with undigested food particles lurking throughout your body. The main thing to remember is that foods fall into different groups (see page 80), and it is important not to eat certain groups at the same time as this will hinder good digestion.

When done properly, food combining will:
► Help your body to burn fat more efficiently
► Ensure the maximum absorption of nutrients, enzymes and proteins
► Prevent burping, bloating, gas and indigestion
► Generally correct or prevent most issues connected with obesity

Without food combining, you:
► Make complete digestion impossible
► Upset digestive enzymes
► Prevent nutrient uptake
► Risk a host of ills, including bloating, heartburn, indigestion, malabsorption, constipation, cramps, irritable bowel syndrome, flatulence or worse

The problem is that some foods are digested more quickly than others; some require different digestive enzymes, and others need different conditions in the stomach for proper absorption. For example, proteins need acid digestive juices, while carbohydrates need alkaline juices for their digestion.

When my own patients embark upon my food-combining methods, they often notice significant improvements in their physical symptoms within just a few days and also report enhanced energy levels, elevated moods and overall vitality.

LOSE THE WEIGHT

Food combining is a great way to manage your weight. The idea is that if you eat a single food by itself, or more than one food in the right combination with other foods, you maximize your digestive capacity and ability to break down the foods effectively. This means your body doesn't hold on to undigested food which then gets turned into fat balls of toxins and cellulite. Proper food combining allows the body to efficiently burn fat. In my practice, I have found proper food combining to be one of the most effective ways to lose and control weight.

HOW IT WORKS

Group 1: Proteins (meat, poultry, cheese, fish, eggs, milk, nuts) produce acid juices for their digestion. They digest slowly.

Group 2: Carbohydrates – these are all grains and the foods made from them (bread, pasta, cereals, flour, biscuits, etc.) and starchy vegetables (such as potatoes, yams and sweetcorn) which produce alkaline juices. They digest quickly and require different enzymes to proteins.

If you eat Groups 1 and 2 together, the competing enzymes and digestive juices will fight and neutralize each other. The result is that food doesn't get digested properly and rots inside the gut, causing gas, bloating, heartburn, stomach pains, malabsorption, indigestion and energy drain, to say the least.

Group 3: Salads, non-starchy vegetables, roots, seeds, herbs, spices, nut and seed oils. These can be digested with either Group 1 or Group 2 above.

Group 4: Fruit. This is out on its own and holds the record for the fastest digestion rate. Fruit uses completely different enzymes from all other groups above.

The Solution:

- Don't eat Group 1 (proteins) and Group 2 (carbohydrates) together at the same meal.
- Group 3 (vegetables) can be eaten with Groups 1 or 2.
- Group 4 (fruit) must always be eaten on its own, at least 30 minutes away from other food groups. It's best to eat fruit on an empty stomach, preferably in the morning with no other food types. If you eat fruit after a meal, it can't go anywhere, because it's stuck behind food that takes much longer to digest, so it will ferment in the gut. When fruit is indeed mixed with other food groups, you can expect bloating, flatulence, indigestion. (Never mix melons with other fruits. Melons digest the fastest of all fruits. Therefore, eat alone or leave alone!)
- Leave 2 hours after a carbohydrate meal before eating protein. Leave 3 hours after a protein meal before eating carbohydrates. Protein takes 4 hours to reach the bowel, and carbohydrate meals take 2 hours from mouth to bowel.

GROUP 1
Proteins
- Cheese
- Eggs (free-range)
- Nuts
- Fish
- Game/rabbit
- Meat
- Milk
- Poultry
- Shellfish
- Soybeans, tofu and all soya products
- Yogurt

GROUP 2
Carbohydrates
- Grains, including oats, pasta, rice, rye, maize, millet
- Grain products, cookies, bread, cakes, crackers and pastry
- Honey
- Maple syrup
- Potatoes and starchy vegetables
- Sugar and sweets

GROUP 3
Non-starchy vegetables
- Salads and fresh herbs
- Seeds
- Butter, cream, spreading fats
- Olive oil (cold-pressed)
- Herbs, spices and seasonings

GROUP 4
- All fruit

Join the path to perfect health. Follow my chart below and improve your digestion, energy and stamina:

FOOD COMBINING CHART

BAD	GOOD
Grain with dairy or meat = gas	Fruit by itself = *no* gas, proper digestion
Fruit with vegetables = gas	Grain with vegetables = *no* gas
Fruit with meats = gas	Pasta with vegetables = *no* gas
Fruit with grain or dairy = gas	Beans with vegetables = *no* gas *
	Fish or meat with vegetables = *no* gas
	Pulses/beans and grains = *no* gas

* Note on beans and grains together: Vegetarians have an easier time when it comes to food combining. Beans have a mixture of starch and protein which may seem a problem. However, starch is dominant in most beans with the exception of soy and navy beans. So, you can combine most beans with grains as well as salads and veggies.

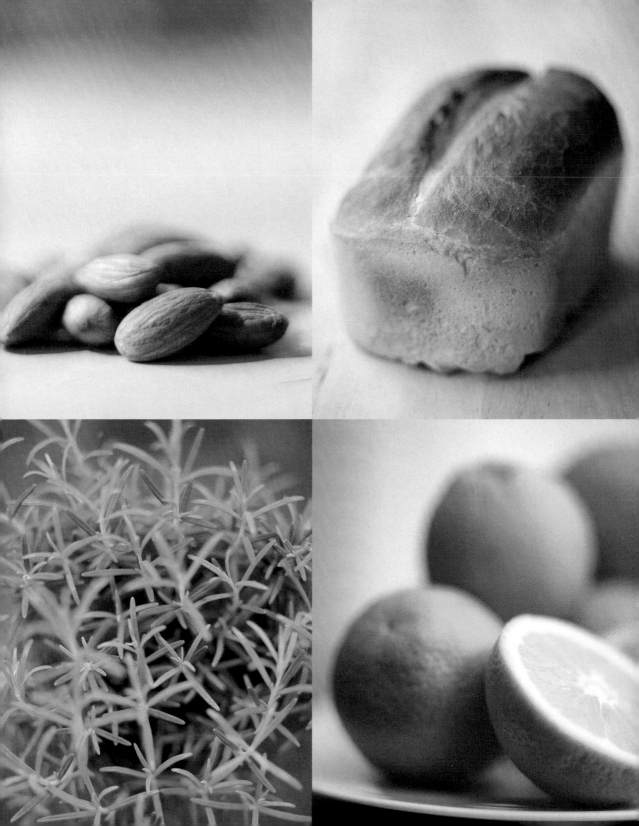

THE ABUNDANT FOOD LIST

Don't let anyone tell you there's nothing left to eat these days. I want you to eat more food than you've ever eaten before. But now you're going to eat the right foods that will keep you slender, fit and lean. And you can eat as much as you want, and you will not get fat or become overweight!

Here is my Abundant Food List. It outlines the Top 100 Foods to eat in your everyday life. And this is just the beginning. If you truly start to eat all of these different foods on a regular basis, I can assure you that you will be doing a grand service to your body, mood and general overall health. As you can see, there is an abundance of many foods that you probably have not been eating or are not even familiar with. Well, now it's time for you to introduce this plethora of foods and start living life to the fullest.

When you adopt my Diet of Abundance, you will feel stronger, sexier, more energized and happier.

LEAFY GREEN VEGETABLES

Beet greens
Chicory
Collards
Dandelion greens
Endive
Escarole
Iceberg lettuce
Kale
Loose-leaf lettuce
Mache
Mustard greens
Turnip greens
Parsley
Rocket
Romaine
Sorrel
Spinach
Swiss chard
Watercress

RAW NUTS

Almonds
Brazil nuts
Cashews (in moderation)
Filberts
Hazelnuts
Chestnuts
Pecans
Pine nuts
Pistachios
Walnuts

SEEDS

Chia
Flax
Pumpkin
Sesame
Sunflower

VEGETABLES

Artichoke
Asparagus
Avocado
Beets
Broccoli
Brussels sprouts
Bok choy
Chinese cabbage
Carrots
Cauliflower
Celeriac
Celery
Daikon
Eggplant
Green peas
Kohlrabi
Okra
Onions
Parsley
Parsnip
Pepper
Potato
Radish
Squash
Tomato
Turnip
Watercress
Yam
Zucchini

FLOURS

Amaranth
Durum wheat
Graham
Oat
Potato
Soy
Sunflower seed
Tapioca

SEA VEGETABLES
(Seaweeds)

Agar
Arame
Dulse
Hijiki
Kelp
Kombu
Nori
Sea palm
Wakame

GRAINS

Amaranth
Barley
Basmati rice
Brown rice
Buckwheat
Bulgur wheat
Corn
Kamut
Millet
Oats
Quinoa
Rye
Spelt

BEANS

Aduki
Anasazi
Black turtle
Fava
Garbanzo
Great northern
Lentils
Lima
Navy
Pinto
Soybeans

FRESH HERBS
(for seasoning)

Basil
Bay
Cardamom
Chervil
Cinnamon
Cloves
Coriander
Cumin
Dill
Fennel
Fenugreek
Ginger
Marjoram
Mint
Oregano
Rosemary
Saffron
Tarragon
Thyme
Umeboshi plums

HERBAL TEAS

Camomile
Dandelion
Fennel
Ginger
Ginseng
Hawthorn
Horsetail
Lemon balm
Licorice
Melissa
Nettle
Pau d'arco
Peppermint
Red clover
Red raspberry
Rose hips
Slippery elm
Spearmint
Valerian root

FRUIT
Cranberries
Currants
Dates
Gooseberries
Grapefruit
Kumquat
Lemons
Limes
Loganberries
Oranges
Passion fruit
Pineapples
Pomegranates
Strawberries
Tangelos
Tangerines

FRUIT
Apples
Apricots
Blackberries
Blueberries
Cherries
Grapes
Guavas
Huckleberries
Kiwi fruits
Loquats
Lychees
Mangos
Mulberries
Nectarines
Papayas
Peaches
Pears
Cactus fruit
i.e. Prickly pears

FRUIT
All dried fruit
Bananas
Dates
Figs
Melons:
Banana melon
Cantaloupe
Honeydew
Watermelon

TOFU

TEMPEH

FISH

People always ask me, "What is the Dr. Gillian McKeith plan in a nutshell?" Here it is: Discover and explore the dozens and dozens of mouthwatering new foods waiting to tantalize your taste buds. Go for it!

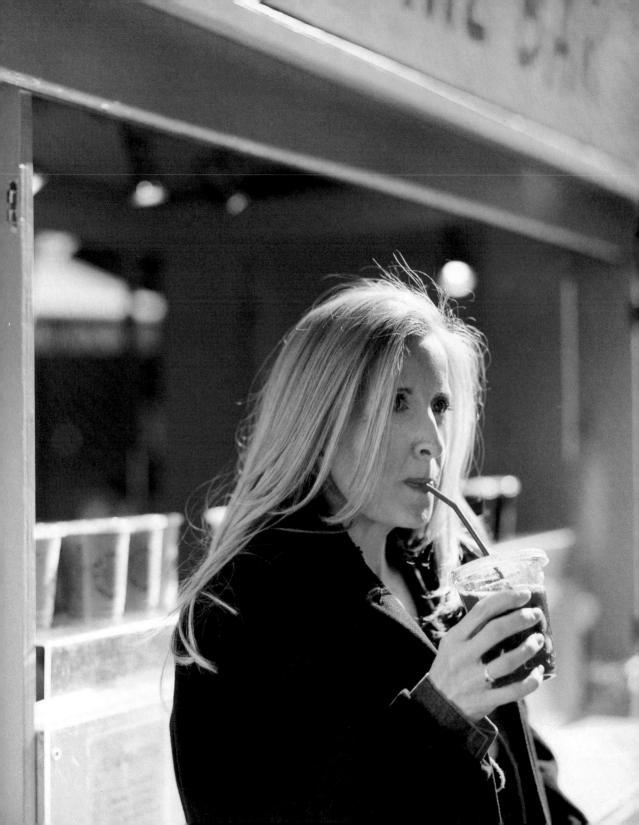

CHAPTER 4

TOP 5 BUMMERS

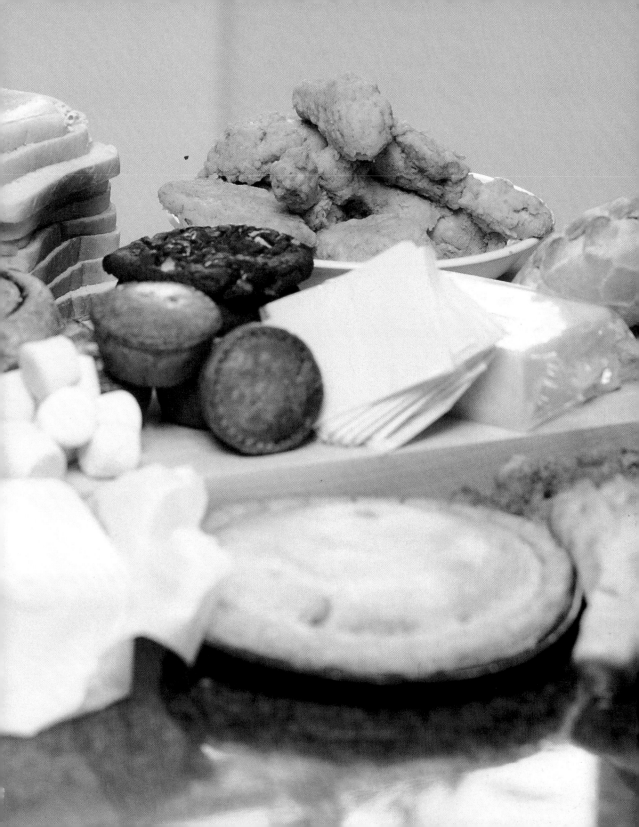

I HAVE FOUND THAT THERE ARE FIVE PROBLEM AREAS INTO ONE OR MORE OF WHICH JUST ABOUT EVERYONE FALLS — AND I CALL THESE "THE BUMMERS." I WOULD SAY THAT ALMOST 95 PERCENT OF MY PATIENTS HAVE A CONDITION THAT FALLS INTO ONE OF THESE CATEGORIES. IF YOU RECOGNIZE ANY OF THESE THEN YOU'LL FIND SOME HELPFUL HINTS FOR EACH IN THIS CHAPTER.

MY TOP 5 BUMMERS:

ALWAYS STRUGGLING WITH WEIGHT
TIRED ALL THE TIME
DIGESTIVE DISORDERS
PMS AND OTHER HORMONAL ISSUES
STRESS

When I saw Yvonne's food diary for the first time, I could not believe how little she ate. Yvonne survived on a diet of potato chips, white bread and chocolate. As a result her body had gone into shutdown mode, causing the metabolism to weaken and the fat-burning mechanism to come to an eventual standstill. And so even though Yvonne didn't eat very much at all, she was really struggling with her weight.

YVONNE'S FOOD DIARY

MONDAY

9am 2 slices white bread, toasted and spread with light margarine
Mug of tea
2pm Large package of chips, package of flavored potato snacks, large chocolate bar, can of diet fizzy drink
11pm Large package of chips, package of flavored potato snacks, large chocolate bar

TUESDAY

9am 2 slices white bread, toasted and spread with light margarine
Mug of tea
11am Coconut and chocolate bar
Cup of hot chocolate
2pm Strawberry meal-replacement milkshake
3pm Microwave pasta, pasta sauce, 2 slices white bread, toasted
6pm Frozen microwave meal – spaghetti Bolognese
Mug of tea
9.30pm 2 slices white bread, toasted and spread with light margarine
Mug of tea

WEDNESDAY

9am 2 slices white bread, toasted and spread with light margarine
Mug of tea
1pm Large baguette filled with creamy Cajun chicken and tomatoes
Bottle of diet cola
3pm Can of ginger ale, package of bacon-flavor chips, package of smokey bacon-flavor chips, package of salted chips, mug of tea
6pm Mug of hot chocolate, 4 fingers of chocolate-covered wafers
7.30pm Half chocolate log cake (about 3–4 portions), mug of tea
9.30pm Pack smokey bacon chips, can of ginger ale, pack of chocolate M&Ms

THURSDAY

8am Package of chips

9am 2 white rolls spread with light margarine and package of chips
Mug of tea

3pm Mug of tea, sponge cake – 2 slices

6pm Individual steak pie, individual chicken and mushroom pie
Can of ginger ale, ½ pack of chocolate beans

FRIDAY

9am Can of ginger ale
2 white rolls spread with light margarine and strawberry jam

12pm 2 packs of cheese-filled crackers, cup of water

5.30pm Mom's homemade curry and rice with pineapple and apple
Mug of coffee

8.30pm 2 packages of chips

9pm Package of chips, mug of coffee, laced with liqueur

SATURDAY

12pm Granola with skim milk

3pm 2 slices white bread, toasted, mug of tea

6.30pm 2 packages of chips

9pm Chinese takeout – sweet 'n' sour Cantonese-style chicken,
egg fried rice, prawn crackers, pint of diet fizzy drink

SUNDAY

9am 2 chocolate biscuits

4pm Can of low-fat soup, 4 slices white bread, package of chips
Mug of tea

8.30pm 2 packages of chips, ½ package of rich tea cookies
2 mugs of tea

ALWAYS STRUGGLING WITH WEIGHT

It is extremely common to be always struggling with weight. You gain weight when the amount of energy taken in from food and drink exceeds the amount of energy used for metabolic processes and exercise. Excess energy is then stored as fat. By following my Diet of Abundance in Chapter 3, you will address all of the following factors which may be currently inhibiting weight loss.

THE WEIGHT-LOSS INHIBITORS

- ► Dirty colon, bowel problems
- ► Eating the wrong foods
- ► Excessive food intake (especially fatty/wrong foods)
- ► Insulin imbalances (caused by too many sugary carbohydrates)
- ► Lack of enzymes
- ► Lack of exercise
- ► Poor digestive function
- ► Mineral and vitamin imbalances
- ► Parasites or worms causing a voracious appetite
- ► Poor adrenal function
- ► Poor eating habits, e.g., not chewing thoroughly, irregular eating times
- ► Poor metabolic function
- ► Sluggish liver
- ► Thyroid problems
- ► Water retention
- ► Weak kidneys
- ► Yeast overgrowth

ARE YOU OVERWEIGHT?

Weight is defined by the Body Mass Index (BMI). To find your BMI, follow calculation below. A BMI of 25 or more is classed as overweight. Over 30 is regarded as obese.

HOW TO CALCULATE YOUR BMI

Multiply your weight in pounds by 704 and then divide by the square of your height in inches.

For example:
126 lbs x 704 ÷ 62^2 = 88704 ÷ 3844 = 23.1
180 lbs x 704 ÷ 69^2 = 126720 ÷ 2761 = 26.6

Check your answer against these ranges:
Underweight below 18.5
Normal 18.5–24.9
Overweight 25–29.9
Obese over 30

STEVIA: CRAVINGS CURBER

You are going to fall in love with this incredible green-leafed plant belonging to the chrysanthemum family. Stevia is a sweet herbal plant that is much sweeter than sugar. But unlike sugar, stevia has the ability to regulate blood sugar levels, suppress sweet cravings and lessen hunger pangs. It's helpful for diabetics and hypoglycemics and contains protein, fiber, complex carbohydrates and vitamins.

To top it all off, stevia has no calories. The glycosides are not metabolized in the body and are thus eliminated without any calories being absorbed. Loads of credible research supports the use of stevia. I use it with patients who have a real sweet tooth. In almost every case, the patient reports a significant decrease or the complete eradication of sugar cravings. It is available in powder or liquid extract.

SUGAR CRAVINGS EXPLAINED

You will crave sugar if your blood sugar levels are constantly out of balance; if you have nutrient deficiencies, yeast overgrowths; if you eat a diet high in refined, processed carbs and junky foods. Sugar cravings are a sign that you may suffer from a condition known as hypoglycemia, causing you to crave even more sugar.

You end up becoming the victim of a seesaw effect of soaring and plummeting sugar levels. This is why if you start to eat just one chocolate bar, you are bound to crave more. The sugar gives you the rush, but this drop is never far behind. The best way to beat the sugar fix is to go cold turkey: no sugary foods or sweets for a month. The herb astragalus can give you a natural energy lift (500mg daily).

You need to support your system with live nutrient-dense superfoods to balance your blood. The superfood spirulina would be a good choice (see page 205). A liquid mineral supplement that contains chromium, manganese and magnesium is important too. Deficiencies of any one of these three minerals cause sugar cravings as blood sugar levels are out of balance. (More than 80 percent of chromium is destroyed in the processing of foods.)

Certain foods help to regulate blood sugar levels and tame sugar cravings. Whole grains and fresh veggies are great choices. Yams, sweet potatoes and squash help to curb a sweet tooth too and they don't elevate blood sugar levels in the way that sugary foods and sweets do.

I often ask my patients to take half a teaspoon of L-Glutamine powder before meals to inhibit food desires. It really helps.

OVEREATING

Parasites or worms in the gut, or emotional issues can make people overeat. (See page 46 for advice on parasites and worms.) And a disruption of organ function or gland imbalances can cause this too. When we eat too much meat, for example, we can inflame the stomach lining which causes an excess of heat in the stomach itself. This heat makes you want to eat more.

FOOD CRAVINGS

Sugary, carbohydrate-rich foods and sweets raise the level of the feel-good chemicals in your body (these are the endorphins serotonin and norepinephrine). The trouble with eating high sugar foods is that sugar enters your bloodstream very quickly and causes a rush of insulin along with a rush of serotonin. If there is a sudden rise in sugar levels, the insulin breaks it down very quickly, leading to a drop in both sugar and endorphins. This leaves you feeling worse than before and you may reach for more sugary foods to boost your mood, setting up a cycle of food cravings, weight gain, fatigue and mood swings which is hard to break. Every single participant on my TV show had a sugar addiction. Most of them did not even realize until I showed them just exactly how much sugar they consumed in a week.

INSULIN IMBALANCES

When you eat food, glucose from the digestive breakdown of the food is absorbed into your gut and blood. The body takes what it requires and then produces insulin to lower glucose levels back to normal, converting the excess glucose into a compound called glycogen which is stored by the liver.

On a healthy diet this process works perfectly, but excessive consumption of refined carbohydrates, particularly sugary foods, upsets the balance and everything starts to go haywire. Your body has to produce increasing amounts of insulin to break down the sugars. Eventually you become resistant to the insulin, and instead of converting excess glucose into glycogen, it turns into fat. You are then caught in a vicious cycle where the more unstable your blood sugar levels, the more prone you will be to craving sweets and unrefined carbohydrates like bread.

An imbalance of the hormone insulin can often be the root cause of overweight. Too much sugar causes glucose intolerance in the body, and when you are overweight you break down sugar less effectively. It's a Catch-22 situation.

GLUCOSE TOLERANCE SELF-CHECK

If you recognize three or more of the symptoms listed below, you may have a problem with the regulation of insulin and glucose in your body.

- ► Difficulty in concentrating
- ► Excessive consumption of caffeine, chocolate or cigarettes
- ► Excessive sweating
- ► Excessive thirst
- ► Extreme difficulty in getting out of bed.
- ► Falling asleep in the middle of the day/feeling really drowsy
- ► Inability to get going without a caffeine/nicotine fix
- ► Irritability without frequent meals
- ► Need for more than eight hours' sleep a night

FOOD INTOLERANCES

We often crave the same foods day in and day out. I had one patient, an artist, who told me that she had to have her oatmeal every morning for breakfast, and only ate breaded chicken legs for dinner every evening for the last thirty years! She was exhausted, no longer wanted to paint, and lacked interest in life. When I forced her to change her same food regimen she became energized, felt creative, started to paint again, and even lost over fifteen pounds in weight within a month.

If you eat the same foods every day, for years, in many cases you can become sensitive to those very foods, conditions sometimes referred to as food intolerances. And usually the foods that we crave are the same ones that lead to weight gain. It is a vicious cycle.

If you are food intolerant, a delayed immune response occurs in your body. This can happen over several hours or days after the offending food is ingested. Side effects to these foods can vary from irritable bowel–like symptoms to skin eruptions, ulcerations in the mouth, Crohn's disease or inflammation of the digestive tract, colic, ear problems and tiredness, to name a few. It is not always so obvious. But food intolerances can have a direct effect on the assimilation of nutrients, digestive organ function and weight management. The more common foods such as wheat, dairy, sugar and corn are often implicated as food intolerance triggers, simply because many of us eat too much of these foods anyway. They can be found in so many prepackaged foods. So it is easy to become food intolerant these days, especially if you eat too many chemically altered and processed foods.

The problem is that when you eat foods to which you are intolerant, every day, you cause a drastic slowdown of metabolism. Digestive enzyme function is impaired, which means that your body will not break down fat properly.

In addition, by eating the same foods every day, you limit your intake of essential nutrients, vitamins, minerals and cofactors. So my best advice here is:

► Always rotate your foods. In other words, if you eat a food today, then try not to eat it again for say three or four days. Thus, you may prevent food intolerances.

► It is a good idea to get tested for food intolerances or allergies. In this way, you can know exactly which foods are possibly causing you to gain weight or feel horrible or overly tired and lethargic. I require all of my weight loss patients, and many other patients too, to get tested at my clinic for food intolerances. Also, do the pulse test (see page 48 for details).

HOW WILL EATING WELL BREAK THE CYCLE?

Eating a balanced, nutrient-rich diet will help you break this cycle of cravings, sugar and weight gain. This is because eating well not only nourishes your body but regulates your blood sugar levels so that you don't get those lows when you crave sugary pick-me-ups. Your energy levels are less likely to dip, which means you are less likely to crave food that you don't need or isn't good for you.

CHRONIC DIETING

Fad diets, or yo-yo dieting, won't help you lose weight in the long term. You may get some short-term weight loss but it will be virtually impossible to sustain. This is because the rate at which food is broken down and used by your body – a process called thermogenesis – is weakened by the stress of constant dieting, making it virtually impossible for you to lose weight and keep it off. Here are my top tips for getting back on track if you have been a chronic dieter:

- Eat a healthy, balanced diet that is high in nutrients.
- Eat widely from my good food list of choices.
- Eat little and often to keep your blood sugar levels stable, reduce food cravings and set you on the right path.
- Choose foods that keep blood sugar levels stable, so anything you like from my Diet of Abundance (page 83). Cut out foods that cause hikes in your sugar levels, particularly sweets and processed foods.
- Get more active. Exercise is an essential long-term weight management tool and ingredient for a healthy, happy life.

- Cut down on salt and drink lots of water to reduce fluid retention (6–8 glasses a day).
- Make breakfast and lunch the biggest meals of the day as you are more likely to be active during the day and burn off the calories.
- The herbs cinnamon, ginger, cayenne, cardamon and ginseng can all help stimulate thermogenesis (the rate at which food is broken down) and promote weight loss.
- Make sure you get enough good quality sleep. Sleep deprivation increases the risk of unhealthy eating and weight gain.
- Motivation:
  - Think about why you want to lose weight and how good it will be for your health and well-being.
  - Start today writing down everything you eat and drink. Once you become more aware of your eating patterns and what triggers food cravings you can start to deal with them.
  - When you do eat take your time. Chew your food really well. Put your knife and fork down between mouthfuls and really savor your food. It takes a while for your stomach to tell your brain that it is full, and many of us eat so fast we never get the signal in time.
  - Write down your weight loss and/or healthy eating goals and make a commitment to yourself. Studies show that writing down your goals helps you stay focused on achieving them.
  - Tell yourself that you are not on a diet. Dieting for a day, a week or a month or a few months belongs to the past. From now on you are simply eating healthily to create a new and exciting you.

Is this you?

▸ Cold hands, and/or feet
▸ Constant headaches
▸ Constipation
▸ Exhaustion, even after sleeping for hours
▸ Feeling cold all the time; taking ages to warm up
▸ Inability to sweat
▸ Infertility
▸ Lethargy in the mornings, while feeling energetic at night
▸ Loss of outer third of eyebrow hair
▸ No desire for sex
▸ Permanent heel cracks
▸ PMS
▸ Swollen eyelids, ankles or hands
▸ Very dry skin and hair
▸ Yellow tint to skin

If you answer yes to three or more of the above questions, you may have an underactive thyroid. Ask your GP for a blood test to check it out. Be aware, however, that sometimes if you have a very mild form of thyroid malfunction, it will go undetected in a blood test.

THE THYROID LINK

The thyroid gland controls the metabolism of your entire body by regulating energy production and oxygen uptake. Continual stress can negatively affect the thyroid gland, depressing its normal function. Overstimulation of the thyroid is caused by the consumption of sugar, coffee and alcohol, sending the thyroid into an exhausted state, which can cause weight gain (especially around your middle, hips and tops of legs) that is very hard to shift.

Solutions:

▸ Kelp supplements can help an underactive thyroid, so can green superfoods (see page 200). Seaweeds which are high in iodine can also help bolster metabolism.
▸ Eat tyrosine-filled food, such as pumpkin seeds, avocados and almonds, to feed your metabolism.
▸ If you are a compulsive eater, taking a tyrosine supplement (500mg, four times a day) along with a zinc supplement (50mg daily) should do the trick.

FOODS RICH IN:

MAGNESIUM	CALCIUM	POTASSIUM
Alfalfa	Broccoli	Apricots
Almonds	Cauliflower	Bananas
Apples	Kale	Carrots
Avocados	Sesame seeds	Cod
Brazil nuts	Split peas	Parsley
Brown rice	Sunflower	Peas
Celery	seeds	Salmon
Dates	Tahini	Sardines
Fish		Spinach
Parsley		Whole grains

NUTRIENT DEFICIENCIES

Nutrient deficiencies may cause weight gain., particularly deficiencies in magnesium, calcium and potassium.

Magnesium deficiencies cause sugar cravings.

Calcium deficiencies inactivate enzymes involved in metabolism. If you are a big meat eater, calcium becomes even more important as high protein diets can create calcium loss.

Potassium deficiencies often occur in overweight people because they drink too much coffee, eat masses of sugar, drink alcohol, use laxatives and diuretics. Potassium helps your heart and regulates water balance in the body. Lowered potassium levels allow the body to harbor excess acids from the residues of bad foods and dietary medications. When potassium levels are normal, the body can attack unwanted acids more efficiently. Excess acids interfere with metabolism and the body's ability to break down foods. When potassium levels are lowered, sodium levels are usually too high. Overweight people with low potassium levels and higher sodium levels usually have too much added table salt in their diets. The more table salt we shake on our foods and the more hidden salt we consume in packaged foods, the more potassium we need.

GILLIAN'S TOP TIPS FOR SHIFTING THE FLAB

▸ Eat early. Late-night eating is a recipe for weight gain because the body stores more food during sleep.

▸ Food combine (see page 78).

▸ Abandon refined or processed foods (see page 26)

▸ Drink 8 glasses of water a day. Water is a natural appetite-suppressant.
Note: Nettle tea is a great weight-loss tea as it supports metabolism and has diuretic properties.

▸ Avoid margarine, full-fat milk, cheeses and cow's milk dairy products. These foods are difficult to digest. You could opt for grain milks instead.

▸ Avoid sugar – it lowers the metabolism.

▸ Cut out wheat (especially bread) because it contains a high level of gluten and many people are intolerant to gluten.

▸ Eat the good fats and throw out the bad. Good fats can be found in avocados, pumpkin seeds, sunflower seeds, fish, nuts and vegetables. Don't avoid these foods. They are high in good fats that fire up your metabolism so that you can lose the weight and keep it off for good. Bad fats are saturated fats, as found in red meats and butter. They are very hard to digest, clog your arteries and lead to illness and weight problems.

▸ Don't skip meals and always eat breakfast. Your stomach and spleen are at their strongest first thing in the morning. You also have the whole day to burn off the meal. If you want to raise metabolism, you have to eat at that time. If you don't, a signal goes to your brain. The brain interprets food as being scarce. Stress hormones are then released

into your body. Muscle tissue is then shed in order to lessen the body's need for food. When you eat later, your body releases more insulin to make more fat as food may be scarce!

▸ Go on my Detox Day (see page 140). Toxins are stored in fatty tissue. It is possible that if you are full of toxins you may have a higher fat-to-muscle ratio. So helping to rid your body of poisons and chemicals can only help improve weight management.

▸ Do not go on fad diets. Dieting slows down the metabolic enzyme function in the body. Your fat cells bloat, become toxic and store in your tissues. You lose muscle tone. You get depressed. Instead, go on my diet of abundance. Eat more than before but the right foods (see page 82).

▸ Exercise. Burn that fat. Exercise raises the metabolic rate so calories are used up faster. To get started, simply start walking – it is a great way to shift fat.

▸ Get your metabolism going. First thing in the morning, drink a cup of warm water with a squeeze of lemon.

▸ Cut out alcohol. It weakens your liver, the basic organ for fat metabolism. Beer and wine are also full of sugar, plus alcohol stimulates your appetite.

▸ Take supplements. All overweight people are deficient in major nutrients. There are also some other helpful nutrients that can help burn fat, increase metabolism and so on. Below I have made a basic list of important nutrients and supplements. I am not suggesting that you take all the supplements I mention all at once.

SUPPLEMENTS FOR WEIGHT LOSS

- *B vitamins* to help metabolize carbs and proteins. Take 50–100mg a day.
- *L tyrosine* to reduce appetite. Take 500mg before all meals.
- *Coenzyme Q10* is a metabolic stimulant that helps facilitate weight loss – especially useful when you're really fatigued. Take 100mg a day.
- *Triphala* to clean out your colon.
- *Superfoods* to fire up your metabolism, provide you with good-quality proteins and balance blood sugars. See page 200.
- *Digestive enzyme supplements* to aid nutrient uptake and help suppress appetite. Take 1 capsule with every meal.
- *Dr. Gillian McKeith Living Food Energy powder* is a great meal replacement when eating on the run.
- *Flax oil supplements or linseeds* to replenish drastically needed EFAs.
- *Chromium polynicotinate* to regulate blood sugar swings. Take 200mcg a day with lunch and dinner.
- *Chickweed* to help break down stubborn fat deposits. Drink 2 cups of chickweed tea a day.
- *Kelp* to support the thyroid gland and weight loss. Take 3 tablets a day or use the seaweed kombu in cooking.
- *Lecithin* to utilize body fats. Take a tablespoon of granules twice a day.
- *Good-quality fiber* to cleanse your system. Take psyllium husks in between meals – with lots of water.
- *Ginseng* to nourish the metabolic system and help the liver to break down fats more effectively. Take 2 tablets daily (500mg) or drink ginseng tea twice daily.

A NOTE ON APPETITE SUPPRESSANTS

I am not in favor of using medications to suppress appetites. There are herbal and nutritional supplements that can play a healthy role in curbing the desire to eat :

- L-5HTP can help appetite suppression. Take 50–100mg twice a day before meals.
- HCA decreases the conversion of sugar into fat and helps curb the hunger pangs (take 500mg twice a day).
- L-Carnitine (an amino acid) helps control sugar levels and raises the metabolism. Take 2000mg a day, divided equally between breakfast, lunch and dinner.

TIRED ALL THE TIME

The single most prominent reason for patients coming to see me is to get more energy. They're tired of feeling tired! You can change all that. You needn't be tired any longer. To maximize energy, we need to include certain foods in our diets, especially those that boost the metabolism and sustain consistent energy levels. The most important nutrients required for energy production are the B complex group of vitamins. Deficiencies in B vitamins can often be the underlying cause of poor adrenal gland function which results in energy slumps. Other metabolism-boosting nutrients include vitamin C, magnesium, zinc, iron, coenzyme Q10 and the herbal plant astragalus.

TOP ENERGY FOODS

SPROUTS – ALL TYPES

All types of sprouts (seeds of legumes or grains that have been germinated) are high-energy, life-enhancing foods that help improve, revitalize, strengthen and regenerate your body. They contain a high concentrate of antioxidants as well as all the trace minerals, plus protein, enzymes and fiber. When seeds are sprouted, their nutritional power swells. See page 213.

GRAINS

Grains release sugar slowly and give you a steady flow of energy instead of a quick high followed by a low. They are also a good source of B vitamins which are needed to assist the spleen, your energy battery. Without the Bs you will definitely need a "jump start."

OATS

Oats are not only packed with energy nutrients but they help keep blood glucose levels at an even keel to maintain concentration and alertness. Enjoy a bowl of porridge in the morning for the perfect release of sustained energy throughout the morning.

PARSLEY

Parsley is a nutrient powerhouse. It contains high levels of vitamin B12, more vitamin C than citrus fruits and just about all other known nutrients.

SEAWEED

Sea vegetables, or seaweeds, are the highest digestible source of all minerals as well as energy-boosting vitamins B and C. See page 208.

VEGETABLES

The range of B complex vitamins, plus the energy nutrients magnesium and iron, can be found in fresh green (preferably raw) vegetables, such as broccoli, asparagus and spinach. Broccoli is also a good source of coenzyme Q10, a critical nutrient for energy production at a cellular level.

PEACHES

Peaches have a high water content and have a laxative effect. They are wonderful in alkalinizing the bloodstream and can be used to regulate the bowel and build the blood. Peaches are one of the best energy fruits because the body assimilates them very easily, giving an instant boost. I often use them in fruit smoothies. They are also great in helping eliminate toxins from the body and are a good food to eat on a weight loss program.

FLAX SEEDS

Flax seeds, or linseeds, contain abundant levels of omega-3 and omega-6 essential fatty acids (EFAs) and in perfect balance. EFAs are involved in energy production and oxygen transfer.

SUNFLOWER SEEDS

The sunflower seed is packed with magnesium, iron, copper, protein, vitamin B complex, EFAs, and zinc. Get into the habit of carrying sunflower seeds around with you for when you need an instant energy pick-me-up.

GRAPES

The therapeutic value of grapes is thought to be due to their high magnesium content. Magnesium is involved in the first stage of the process that converts energy to glucose.

YAMS AND SQUASHES

Yams are packed with energy minerals and loads of vitamin C. Yams are also detoxifying and balancing to hormone and blood sugar levels, ensuring that your energy supply is constant. Squashes motivate the circulation of energy meridians, especially strengthening digestive function.

WHEATGRASS

Wheatgrass is a rich nutritional food that looks like grass and contains one of the most prolific arrays of vitamins, minerals and trace elements. It contains twenty-five times the nutrients of your choicest vegetables. See page 203.

MUNG BEANS

To feel full of beans means you are bursting with energy. And that's just what mung beans can provide you with: bags of energy.

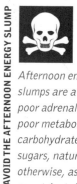

AVOID THE AFTERNOON ENERGY SLUMP

Afternoon energy slumps are a sign of poor adrenal function, poor metabolism of carbohydrates and sugars, natural or otherwise, as well as nutrient-depleted foods. Reduce your intake of sugar, caffeine and dairy foods at lunch and opt instead for brown rice, legumes, yams and sunflower seeds. Snack on sprouted seeds too for a quick pick-me-up. You can also feed your adrenals with the B vitamins. Take a B complex, 50mg at lunchtime. I drink cups of hot water with herbal tinctures of astragalus and ginseng for my afternoon lifts, a natural source of the B vitamins.

DIGESTIVE DISORDERS

IT'S NORMAL TO PASS WIND NOW AND AGAIN,
BUT EXCESSIVE GAS, SMELLY STOOLS AND
HEARTBURN ARE SIGNS OF POOR DIGESTIVE
FUNCTION, NUTRIENT DEPLETION, PUTRID
INTESTINAL BACTERIAS, LAZY BOWEL AND
STOMACH FUNCTION. THESE CAN LEAD TO ALL
KINDS OF HEALTH PROBLEMS IF LEFT UNCHECKED.

CONSTIPATION

You need to empty out your bowels approximately twice a day, regularly and without effort. Any less than once a day and you are very likely constipated. Difficult bowel movements such as sitting on the toilet for ages, trying to force something out, or dropping little "rabbit pellets" are also signs that you may be constipated. Follow my dietary guidelines below if you are suffering from constipation.

REDUCE
- Dairy products
- Meats
- Saturated fats
- Spicy or hot foods
- Sugar and sweets
- Tea and coffee

INCREASE
- Fresh fruits (eat fruit in the morning by itself, not with other food groups, see page 78)
- Green vegetables
- Sprouted seeds
- Whole grains
- Have plenty of rest
- Drink plenty of fluids
- Exercise moderately
- Eat slowly and chew your food thoroughly

ONGOING CONSTIPATION SUPPORT
- Eat raw sauerkraut.
- Beneficial bacteria in the form of acidophilus (1 or 2 capsules a day).
- One digestive enzyme supplement with every meal.
- Linseeds and pumpkin seeds (2 tablespoons of linseeds ground with 1 tablespoon of pumpkin seeds). Eat with a salad and chew really well. Alternate with a tablespoon of black sesame seeds.

ANTI-CONSTIPATION SUPPLEMENT PROGRAM
- Aloe vera, 1 tablespoon twice daily (mix with apple juice if preferred)
- Triphala, 1 teaspoon in glass of water or juice, 1 hour before bed
- Wild blue-green algae or spirulina, 2 teaspoons daily or 2 tablets a day
- Flax oil, 1 capsule or 1 teaspoon a day
- Psyllium husks, 1 teaspoon in 10oz glass of water or juice
- Milk thistle, 1 capsule or 20 drops of liquid tincture in water three times a day
- Vitamin C with bioflavonoids, 1000mg, three times a day
- Vitamin B Complex (rice based), 25–50mg, twice a day with meals
- Magnesium, 400mg, three times a day

HERBS FOR CONSTIPATION
- Cascara sagrada (for short-term relief)
- Senna (for short-term relief)
- Barberry
- Rhubarb root
- You will also be able to find herbal formulas specifically for constipation in your local health food store

- Teas:
- Nettle tea: 3 cups daily is a great bowel wakener
- Slippery elm

It is normal to have occasional gas. But continual wind, bloating and/or flatulence are not the norm. Junky diets, too much sugar, wheat and dairy make the problem worse.

Solutions

- Drink liquids 20–25 minutes *before* meals, or one hour after meals. Don't drink liquids with your meals.
- Eat dinner early. Eating late at night depletes the stomach of fluids at a time when its energy is at its weakest. You will end up with indigestion and will not absorb nutrients properly.
- Food combine. See page 78
- Eat when you're relaxed. Total relaxation while eating renders maximum digestion. There's no point in eating if you are angry, upset or emotional.
- Drink 1 tablespoon of aloe vera juice and a teaspoon of liquid chlorophyll before your largest meal to stimulate digestion.
- Take a digestive enzyme supplement with meals. See page 209.
- Use herb seasonings (e.g. dill, fennel, thyme and mint) to reduce gas in the gut. Don't use salt, which hampers protein digestion and absorption of nutrients. Use seaweed seasonings instead.
- Eat slowly and chew thoroughly.
- Eat smaller meals.
- Miso soup, whole grains, fresh veggies and fruits are all good for flatulence.
- Drink peppermint and fennel teas.
- Take digestive enzymes with every meal to break down foods and an acidophilus supplement daily to help restore good bacteria in your gut.

IRRITABLE BOWEL SYNDROME

The symptoms of irritable bowel syndrome (IBS) are unpleasant and varied but are often a combination of tummy pain, bloating, cramping, constipation and diarrhea. An additional sign is mucus in your stools.

Many people blame stress for IBS. Certainly, stress can induce gastrointestinal spasms, but the main cause is likely to be what I call a "backup" in your body's "plumbing system" – which means your digestive system is under too much strain and your intestines do not work properly. This results in an erratic quality to the strength of contractions which move your food waste through the intestinal tract. When the contractions are too fast and strong, you get diarrhea; when they are too slow, you become constipated. You also end up quite depleted nutritionally as this condition interferes with the absorption of nutrients.

Note: IBS can be mistaken for a more serious condition such as ulcerative colitis, diverticulitis or Crohn's disease, so please consult your doctor.

THE NO-NOS

- Cut out wheat, cheese, dairy, eggs, corn, processed foods, sugars, sweeteners, margarine, red meat, alcohol and coffee for two months and monitor the results. You may have overburdened your system with the glutens and mucus from these foods.
- Do not overeat, and chew your food really well. It's a good idea to drink veggie juices once a day. See page 145 for ideas.
- Eat a high-fiber diet of whole grains, vegetables, legumes and sprouted seeds (see page 212). These pass smoothly through the intestinal tract.
- However, go easy at first on broccoli, cauliflower, onions and cabbage, which may aggravate this condition.

Supplements:
- Take protein digestive enzymes.
- 2 tablespoons flax oil daily.
- Sprinkle 1 tablespoon linseeds over salads.
- 1 tablespoon aloe vera juice before meals to calm down inflammation in the gut.
- B complex, 50mg daily, to help you break down your foods as well as act as a digestive enzyme supplement with meals.
- 1000mg twice daily of L-Glutamine powder can do wonders.
- Triphala tablets and milk thistle tincture, 15 drops, three times daily helps too. Drink pau d'arco teas.
- A good 6 months on an intestinal probiotic powder or capsule is beneficial too.

Herbs:
- The best one for this condition is gentiana root (available from health food stores). Thirty drops in water before all meals should do the trick.
- Peppermint oil capsules are helpful too. Follow directions on the package.

INDIGESTION

This is usually caused by heavy consumption of greasy or spicy foods or eating too much, too fast. It's normal to pass wind now and again, but excessive flatulence and burping, smelly stools and heartburn are signs of poor digestive function, nutrient depletion, putrid intestinal bacterias, lazy bowel and stomach function. These can lead to all kinds of health problems if left unchecked.

Here are some solutions:

▶ Pear and peach juice – 2 pears and 2 peaches put through the juicer and sipped slowly will do wonders. A dash of powdered ginger and a squeeze of lime can help too.

▶ Banana blend juice – blend a banana with pear or mango juice. It is smooth, easy to digest and will relieve your stomach inflammation.

And to help prevent it:

▶ Take L-Glutamine (1 teaspoon before meals).

▶ Avoid heavily spiced foods, junky foods, fried foods, caffeine, alcohol, fizzy drinks, rich creamy foods, full-fat cheeses or wheat-based foods.

▶ Apple cider vinegar is a wonderful digestive tonic. Add 1–2 teaspoons to a little warm water and sip slowly before meals.

▶ Drink fennel, catnip, slippery elm, peppermint, camomile or thyme teas.

Note: Commercial antacids neutralize stomach acid but over the long term can lead to your stomach producing even more acid. And many antacids contain aluminium, which leaches calcium from your bones.

EAT FOODS TO SUPPORT THE LIVER

Since the liver must process the by-products of whatever we eat, make the job easy. Eating the right foods is crucial here. Eat unprocessed foods as much as possible. Quickie, prepackaged foods laden with chemicals, preservatives, colorings and flavorings overwork the liver. Cakes, sugary cookies, processed, refined or fried foods lack nutrients and are improperly absorbed, further weakening the liver. Instead, eat more of the following food groups, which are specifically nourishing to the liver and liver function:

DRINKS

Eliminate fizzy drinks as they interfere with digestion. Many are loaded with phosphates that deplete the body of vital minerals. Drink fresh water and juices instead.

FRUITS

Certain fresh fruits help to stimulate energy flow through the liver, especially dark grapes, blackberries, huckleberries, strawberries, blueberries and raspberries. (Note: Always eat fruit by itself, preferably in the morning.)

GRAINS, VEGETABLES AND LEGUMES

Include foods which balance the flow of emotional and physical liver energy: grains, vegetables and legumes. Some of these foods tend to contain a slight natural sweetness; but it's a good sweet which harmonizes the liver. The natural inclination for a tired or stressed mom is to reach for a quick high-sugar fix though – cookies, cakes, ice cream, chocolate. When you feel that desire for high-sugar sweets coming on, opt for a sweet vegetable such as a yam or sweet potato. Sweet potato and squash soup can curb many a craving. Also, train yourself to indulge in some of the following:

FOODS WITH SULFUR

Sulfur-containing vegetables are high in specific liver building enzymes. Therefore, include generous amounts of:

► Broccoli
► Nuts
► Brussels sprouts
► Seeds (especially flax, sunflower and pumpkin)
► Cabbage
► Kohlrabi
► Cauliflower
► Turnip roots

LECITHIN

Sprinkle lots of Lecithin granules over salads. Lecithin helps the liver.

GRAINS
► Amaranth
► Millet
► Quinoa

VEGETABLES
► Asparagus
► Basil
► Bay leaves
► Beets
► Black pepper
► Cardamom
► Celery
► Cucumber
► Cumin
► Daikon radish
► Dill
► Fennel
► Garlic

LEGUMES
► Kidney beans
► Peas
► Soybeans
► Tofu

► Ginger
► Lemon
► Mustard greens
► Onions
► Red beets
► Radish
► Radish leaves
► Romaine lettuce
► Rosemary
► Seaweeds
► Umeboshi plums
► Watercress

PMS AND OTHER
HORMONAL ISSUES

Period pain, angry moods and PMS can play havoc with your life.
I used to feel like the "Queen of Periods from Hell." Without fail, at
that time of the month, I was a basket case: migraines, cramps, swelling,
bloating, engorged breasts, fever, nausea, vomiting. Luckily it is now
a thing of the past.

Once I was invited to attend the American Health Foods Industry
Conference. This was a large national exhibition, where all the natural
health companies came to display their wares. Before giving my talk,
I decided to roam the convention hall where there were hundreds of
different companies displaying healthy products. There was one problem,
however. I was in the midst of my monthly menstrual cycle. And yes, it
was the "Mother of all Periods"! As I entered one booth, I was suddenly
overcome with intense nausea and dizziness. Everything began to spin.

Then I fainted. I lost consciousness right in the middle of one of the
busiest locations at the nation's largest natural health convention. As
I came to, dozens of natural food retailers and health food manufacturers
were standing above me while I lay on the floor. One man was screaming
for a doctor, another person was hollering for smelling salts. And all
I could think was, "Calm down boys, it's just my monthly period."

SO HERE ARE MY FEW TIPS FOR AN EASIER TIME

1 Take the herb milk thistle (2 capsules three times a day), four days before and during menstruation. Milk thistle protects the liver and helps normalize estrogen levels. If you do nothing else, take this supplement.

2 Decongest your liver with the use of lipotropic agents. Lipotropics quicken the removal of fat deposits and bile. Simply stated, they "decongest" the liver, improving organ function and assisting metabolization of fats. PMS has been linked to faulty liver fat metabolism. A good liver formula should consist of approximately 1000mg of choline, 500mg of methionine and/or cysteine.

3 Deficiencies of either magnesium or zinc will affect liver function. For example, a deficiency of magnesium results in increased lead absorption. Most patients I see suffering from PMS have low magnesium and/or zinc levels, and high lead or heavy metal toxicity. Magnesium deficiency is strongly implicated as a contributing factor to premenstrual syndrome. The zinc is important because it helps normalize hormones. Take approximately 1200mg magnesium and 50mg zinc daily.

4 Increase your intake of B vitamins, including B6 (a magnesium deficiency can lead to decreased B vitamin activity). Do not use isolated B6; instead, take B6 with a B complex or from botanical royal jelly. Take 50–100mg B complex every day, or 2 capsules of royal jelly three times a day.

5 Vitamin A has been shown to reduce PMS symptoms. Take approximately 10,000iu daily in beta-carotene form. Do not take supplements of vitamin A if you are pregnant.

6 Vitamin E in double-blind studies has demonstrated a reduction in physical symptoms of PMS as it regulates hormone levels. Take 400iu a day.

7 Take 1 tablespoon of flax oil or evening primrose oil or borage oil every day. Women with menstrual problems have been shown to exhibit essential fatty acid abnormalities.

8 The following herbs may be helpful a couple of days before and during:
Ongoing: agnus castus – breast pain and hormonal balance
Rotate: angelica dong quai – cramps
cramp bark – abdominal discomfort
licorice – water retention
black cohosh – fibroids
If you had to choose just one of the above, then opt for the agnus castus. It can work wonders.

9 Eat the right foods as outlined in this book. Cut out the milky products at least ten days prior to period onset. This can make all the difference. Use a complete superfood such as spirulina, wild blue-green algae or chlorella, along with royal jelly. You should increase the intake of these superfoods as the period nears.

10 Regular moderate exercise throughout the month helps regulate hormones, removes toxins, enhances nutrient absorption, strengthens the organs and ultimately lessens PMS symptoms.

MENOPAUSAL SOLUTIONS

A healthy, fully functioning liver is crucial for good health during menopause. It provides vital energy for all the body systems, helps regulate digestion, assists the release of toxins and waste, improves metabolism, balances hormones and nourishes hair, skin, nails, eyes and cells. Menopausal women tend to be low in substances and fluids which nurture the liver, and it is absolutely crucial during this time of hormonal flux that the liver is properly nourished and supported.

Strengthen the liver with the liver building foods on page 108 and the supplements outlined below, and your menopausal symptoms will either disappear or be dramatically reduced.

FOODS FOR THE MENOPAUSE

► Apples
► Aduki beans
► Fennel
► Flax seeds
► Kidney beans
► Oats
► Olives
► Sesame seeds
► Soybeans
► Split peas
► Sunflower seeds
► Yams

► Drinking sage tea (2 cups a day), or 15 drops of sage tincture in a small amount of water, can do wonders for hot flashes and related menopausal symptoms. Black cohosh (40mg a day) has also been shown to diminish hot flashes through the production of estrogen.
► The homeopathic remedy Lachesis 12c is helpful too.
► Agnus castus, also known as vitex, can rebalance hormones by helping to produce more progesterone. It works for menstrual women and it can work for you too. Take this in combination with the herb donq quai for maximum effect.
► The supplement DHEA (10mg a day) is helpful. It's an adrenal hormone that can increase estrogen levels. As you get older, production of DHEA declines.
► The herb red clover, high in B vitamins, and the supplement gamma oryzenol have made positive changes with my patients. All of these supplements are available in health food stores. Don't be afraid to ask for them.
► Natural progesterone cream from wild yam has been shown to make some improvement in menopausal symptoms. It contains naturally occurring DHEA.

STRESS

Everybody tells me that they are stressed. Stress rears its ugly head everywhere: in the workplace, at home, in our personal relationships, and even in the kitchen through the poor food some may eat.

Stress is the manifestation of how we handle our life episodes. Some people are innately and genetically better at dealing with stress. Others can train and teach themselves to handle stress more efficiently. The right food choices can dramatically assist the body in better handling stress. Therefore, we have more control over stress than we might realize. Nonetheless, the bottom line is that stress causes a pumping out of toxic substances in the bloodstream which makes you tired, irritable and angry. Stress also depletes the body of vitamins, minerals and other nutrients. It degrades digestive function and slows the metabolism, which leads to weight gain.

The good news, however, is that you *can* do something. We can reduce our reactions to stress. We can also enhance our lifestyle to improve biochemistry and physiology to better deal with the stress. Instead of eating junk foods when you get stressed, you can choose healthy de-stress foods that will calm your body down. See my list on pages 118–120 for the "De-Stress Foods" to keep you calm and relaxed.

STRESS SELF-CHECK

By taking my self-check test here you will be able to determine your stress levels. Answer "YES" or "NO" to the following questions:

IS THIS YOU?

Constant tiredness?

Immense slump in middle of day?

Spare tire around the middle?

Constant cravings for bread or pasta?

Cravings for salt or sweets?

Mood swings?

Angry? Irritable?

Bloated after eating?

Exhausted upon waking?

Depressed or feeling blue?

Jumpy? Restless?

Apathetic? Can't be bothered?

Insomnia?

Indigestion? Gas? Flatulence?

Prolonged emotional stress?

Drink lots of stimulant drinks?

Food allergies and chemical sensitivities?

Crave alcohol?

Always hungry?

Heart palpitations? Flutters?

Headaches?

Cry easily?

Constipated or diarrhea?

Fungal infections?

Light-headed? Dizziness?

Premenstrual tension?

Hair loss?

Brown pigment spots?

Inability-to-cope feeling? (It's all too much)

Difficulty relaxing or switching off?

SCORING

If you answered yes to less than five of the above questions, then you may be cool as a cucumber and you win my De-Stress Self-Check Test.

If you answered yes to between five and nine of the above questions, then you are feeling a bit stressed out and you certainly would benefit from following my recommendations.

If you answered yes to ten or more of the above questions, then you really are stressed high as a kite. You need to start following my advice immediately – you will soon feel the benefits.

FIGHT OR FLIGHT

The initial response to stress is the alarm reaction, often referred to as the fight or flight response. This is triggered by reactions in the brain that cause the pituitary gland (the master gland of your body's entire hormonal system) to send chemical messages to the adrenal gland to secrete adrenaline and other stress-related hormones.

The fight or flight response is designed to help you deal with danger. The muscles, heart, lungs and brain are given priority fuel, and all other bodily systems are subdued. Your heart rate increases, oxygen and glucose are sent in increased amounts to your muscles, and you'll notice that you breathe faster and you sweat to lower your body temperature. Your blood sugar also goes up as your liver dumps stored glucose into the bloodstream and your adrenal gland pumps out stress hormones, such as adrenaline, to keep the fight or flight reaction going.

All these and many other complex changes occur, some of them in a split second. They all serve one purpose: to gear you up for immediate action or to sharpen your responses in a crisis; for example, your quick response when you grab your child just as he or she tries to run into a busy road. When the danger is over, the biochemicals of stress are used up as intended and the body adapts to normal stress and equilibrium. No harm is done.

HAVOC WITH YOUR HORMONES

The trouble is when the stress is prolonged because it is caused by something you can't immediately deal with or do much about – a delayed train, screaming children, the phone ringing, the ATM machine swallowing your card, being late for an appointment, a frustrating meeting or job. Instead of the stress reaction being short-lived, it persists for long periods of time and when this happens, it can have profound effects on your body. Your body stays in this heightened state of alert, adrenaline continues to pump around your body and your hormones can't return to their normal state.

The hormonal chaos prolonged stress causes can increase your risk of blood sugar problems, high blood pressure, fatigue, adrenal exhaustion and weight gain.

FOODS THAT STRESS

A well-balanced diet is crucial in preserving health and helping to reduce stress. Certain foods and drinks act as powerful stimulants to the body and hence are a direct cause of stress. This stimulation can overwork the liver, upset blood sugar levels and be harmful in the long run.

▸ Caffeine. This is found in coffee, tea, chocolate, cola, etc. It causes the release of adrenaline, thus increasing the level of stress. Caffeine addicts wear out the stress hormone–producing adrenal glands. These stress hormones interfere with metabolism. So caffeine will cause weight gain in the long term, especially if combined with a poor diet. Consuming too much caffeine has the same effect as long-term stress.

▸ Alcohol is a major cause of stress. The irony is that most people take to drinking as a way to combat stress. Alcohol and stress, in combination, are quite deadly. Alcohol stimulates the secretion of adrenaline, resulting in problems such as nervous tension, irritability and insomnia. Excess alcohol will increase the fat deposits in the heart and decrease the immune function. Alcohol also limits the ability of the liver to remove toxins from the body. During stress, the body produces several toxins. In the absence of their filtering by the liver, these toxins continue to circulate through the body, resulting in serious damage.

▸ Sweets. Sugar has no essential nutrients. It provides a short-term boost of energy through the body, resulting possibly in the exhaustion of the adrenal glands. This can result in irritability, poor concentration, and depression. High sugar consumption puts a severe load on the pancreas. There is increasing possibility of developing diabetes.

▸ Salty foods. Salt increases the blood pressure, depletes adrenal glands and causes emotional instability. Use a salt substitute that has potassium rather than sodium. Avoid processed foods high in salt, such as bacon, ham, pickles, sausages, etc.

▸ Fatty foods. Avoid the consumption of foods rich in saturated fats, such as animal foods, dairy products, fried foods and common junk foods. Fats put unnecessary stress on the cardiovascular system.

▸ Cow's milk and dairy products. These stress the body because they contain substances, such as the protein casein, that are difficult and unsuitable for humans to digest and can trigger allergic responses.

▸ Red meat. High-protein red meat elevates brain levels of dopamine and norepinephrine, both of which are associated with higher levels of anxiety and stress.

▸ Refined and processed foods, such as white refined bread and flour, stress the body because they are low in nutrients and high in empty calories. Moreover, in order to digest refined foods your body has to use its own vitamins and minerals, so depleting its stores. Foods containing white flour include cakes, cookies, bread and pastries.

- Margarines and other processed vegetable oils. These are high in trans-fatty acids and a diet too high in trans-fatty acids can have a negative effect on cholesterol, increasing the risk of heart disease. They can also block the body's assimilation of health-boosting essential fatty acids.
- Spicy foods. Spices contain volatile oils which are capable of physically irritating the lining of the stomach. Hot curries, chilies and chili sauces used in Mexican and Indian foods and some drinks are best avoided. A very hot chili or curry dish that contains a blend of pungent spices can literally bore a hole in the stomach lining.
- Additives, preservatives and other chemicals. Additives place a huge stress on your body because your body has to work harder to deal with them, with the result that energy and valuable nutrients are spent when they could be used more profitably, for example in boosting the immune system.

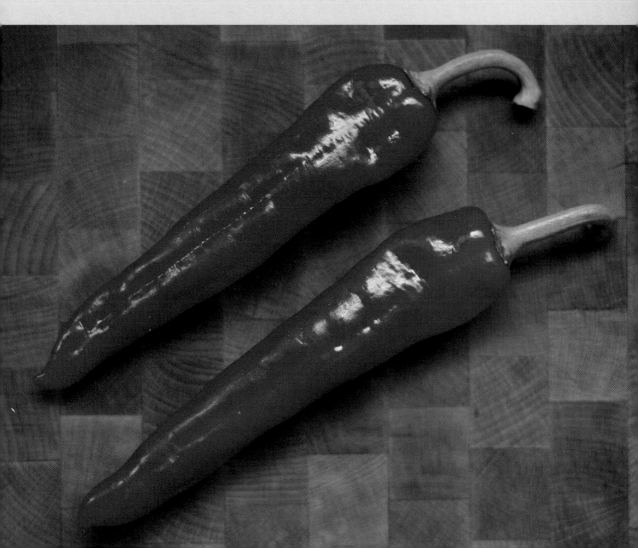

FOODS THAT DE-STRESS

Your body responds to stress with increased production of adrenal stress hormones, and these hormones are responsible for many of the symptoms we associate with stress: elevation of blood pressure, muscle tension, digestive upsets, etc. Overproduction of adrenal stress hormones can also lead to nutritional deficiencies and an exhausted adrenal gland. When the adrenal gland is exhausted, this can alter your response to stress and lead to chronic exhaustion and anxiety. Because of the importance of the adrenal gland for proper nutrition and the stress response, nutrient-rich foods that support adrenal gland function are particularly beneficial for stress reduction.

▸ Celery. An old folk remedy to lower blood pressure. I recommend 2–4 celery stalks daily to my stressed-out patients. Compounds within the celery lower the concentrations of stress hormones that cause blood vessel constriction. Celery contains nutrients that calm, including niacinimide. A stalk of celery before bedtime may even improve your sleep.

▸ Sunflower seeds. Not only are sunflower seeds a rich source of potassium, they are also rich in B vitamins (in particular B6 and pantothenic acid) and zinc which play a critical role in the health of the adrenal glands. Evidence suggests that during times of stress the levels of these nutrients can plummet.

▸ Brown rice is a slowly absorbed carbohydrate that can help trigger the release of the body's feel-good chemicals, serotonin and norepinephrine. It can help you deal better with stress by helping to lift your mood and giving you a more sustained burst of energy.

▸ Algae. The body's feel-good hormones, serotonin and norepinephrine, can also be made from tryptophan and L-phenylalanine, amino acids present in certain protein foods. Algae contains approximately 60 percent protein and is derived from all eight essential amino acids. Algae exerts an energetic effect on the liver and can help to facilitate the elimination of toxins, thus lowering stress levels in the body. Algae contains virtually every nutrient known to man, including all those that have a positive effect on the nervous system. It provides the essential nutrients that stress will rob from the body. You can buy algae in a health food store.

▸ Cabbage is a good stress-busting source of the antioxidant vitamins A, C and E, beta-carotene and the mineral selenium. Antioxidants fight the damaging effect of free radicals in your body released in response to stress and they also help the conversion of tryptophan to serotonin, thus playing their part in boosting mood.

▸ Almonds are rich in magnesium which is especially important for supporting adrenal function as well as the metabolism of essential fatty acids. Low levels of magnesium can be associated with nervous tension, anxiety, irritability and insomnia. Almonds are a great source of magnesium (soak them overnight for easy digestion).

▸ Berries. Blackberries are rich in manganese and vitamin C. Insufficient vitamin C can weaken your immune system and make you feel generally stressed and run down. Other good food sources of vitamin C and manganese include strawberries and raspberries.

- Sesame seeds. The need for zinc increases during times of stress, and it is important for the metabolism of fatty acids and for the production of serotonin. Sesame seeds are a good food source of zinc.
- Cucumbers. The old saying "keeping cool as a cucumber" is literally true because of its cooling effect on the blood and the liver. When the liver is properly nourished and not overheated, this critical organ can help to balance hormones, boost mood, beat stress and deliver vibrant health. Try drinking cucumber and celery juice.
- Asparagus. Many of the elements that build the liver, kidneys, skin, ligaments and bones are found in green asparagus. It also helps in the formation of red blood capsules, and is also high in the antioxidant enzyme glutathione which helps the liver function at optimum levels. Anything that has a positive effect on your liver has a positive effect on your mood and your ability to deal with stress.
- Garlic. This has been used throughout history to treat colds and flu and for feeling generally run-down; now folklore has been backed up by science. Garlic contains a detoxifying chemical called allicin, which is responsible for its characteristic taste and smell. When you can get rid of circulating toxins, you feel less stressed. Garlic can also have a huge impact on the lowering of blood pressure associated with stress. A powerful antibiotic, allicin has both antiviral and antifungal powers as well as cholesterol-lowering, blood pressure–lowering and mood-boosting effects.
- Avocados. These contain 14 minerals, all of which regulate body functions and stimulate growth. Especially noteworthy is their iron and copper content which aids in red blood regeneration and the prevention of nutritional anemia – one very common cause of fatigue and inability to cope effectively with stress.

Herbal teas can be very effective at relieving many stress symptoms. These teas are derived from the flowers, leaves, seeds, stalks, stems and roots of plants. They contain natural substances that nourish the central nervous and glandular systems. Give them a try. Find which ones works best for you.

- Camomile
- Ginseng
- Hops
- Kava
- Lemon balm
- Licorice
- Oatstraw
- Passionflower
- Skullcap
- Valerian

HERBS TO HELP YOU COPE

My patients have reported great results using the following.

- *Eleutherococous senticosus,* commonly known as Siberian ginseng (100–500mg a day). Siberian ginseng and panax ginseng increase the tone and function of the adrenal glands, helping to balance the hormonal excretions. Ginseng has been shown in studies to protect against the effects of physical and mental stress. *Note: Do not use extracts of panax (Chinese) or American ginseng if you have high blood pressure.*
- Licorice root (70mg capsules or 15 drops of a 5:1 liquid extract three times a day). Licorice is most beneficial for correcting low cortisol output and will give the adrenal glands a chance to rest and recover.
- Rhodiola increases the body's natural resistance to stressors.
- Astragalus supports the immune system and helps the body adapt to stress (500mg, once or twice daily).

VITAMINS AND MINERALS

Your body's levels of these key nutrients plummet during times of stress. Try the following anti-stress package to be taken daily:

- 1000–2000mg vitamin C (choose one which contains bioflavonoids for extra protection)
- 300mg magnesium
- 200mg calcium
- 500mg vitamin B5 (pantothenic acid)
- Mega B complex (choose one which contains around 75mg of each of the major B vitamins)
- Antioxidant formula (pick a brand containing about 25,000iu beta carotene, 200iu vitamin E, 30mg zinc and 200mcg selenium)
- 100–500mg tyrosine (an amino acid) twice a day when under significant prolonged stress
- Or take a multivitamin powder

POOR IMMUNITY IMMUNE SYSTEM SELF-CHECK

Is this you?

A diet high in processed and/or sugary foods

Allergies or food sensitivities

Amalgam dental fillings (which contain mercury)

Close family members with a degenerative illness

Exposure to poor-quality air on a daily basis

Feeling tired or under the weather most of the time

Frequent colds or flu

Gastrointestinal problems

Lack of exercise

Less than eight hours' sleep a night/Insomnia

Living in or near a major city or a busy street

Living near high-voltage power lines, cell phone towers or a nuclear power plant

Living under constant stress

Recurring thrush or yeast infections

Regular consumption of tap water, fizzy drinks or sodas

Signs of premature aging

Smoking and/or drinking alcohol frequently

Teethmarks or scalloped edging round the sides of your tongue

Using a computer or cell phone every day

Using a microwave oven regularly

The more questions you answer yes to, the more impaired your immune system is likely to be.

TOP 5 BUMMERS

IMMUNE BOOSTERS

SPROUTED BROCCOLI SEEDS
See page 213 on how to grow in your kitchen. Scientists have discovered that sprouted broccoli seeds contain 30–50 times more active and more absorbable levels of specific antioxidant immune properties than regular non-sprouted broccoli. (Regular broccoli is still really good for you, though, and I highly recommend it.) Sprouted broccoli seeds are high in sulforophane, a powerful antioxidant. They boost long-lasting immune support. Eat these sprouts twice weekly.

ASTRAGALUS
500mg twice daily provides an immunity tonic which maintains our defences. This super herbal food raises the body's resistance to external pathogens and strengthens your body's effectiveness in fighting viruses and infections.

GINSENG ROOT
Ginseng is a nutritive tonic. It neutralizes the effects of free radicals (destructive molecules) during periods of stress. It sends messages through the immune system, acting as a catalyst for the release of certain hormones essential for immune defence.

REISHI AND SHIITAKE MUSHROOMS
Use in soups, stews and as a side dish. These incredible mushrooms are a natural source of a protein which induces immune response. They contain a compound called lentinal which mobilizes our natural defenses, and protect the body by lowering heat toxins created from overly acid diets. They are also an excellent source of the antoxidant germanium which supports your immune system.

OREGON GRAPE
Easily obtainable from a health food store, it contains a compound called berberine which supports the fight against nasty bacteria.

OLIVE LEAF
This herb contains an effective natural antibiotic support against dozens of bacteria strains.

GINGER ROOT
Ginger nurtures the regulation of compounds important for immunity. It has a soothing, antiseptic support action on the body's ability to handle external wind and cold.

LICORICE ROOT
This herb and tea helps to counteract the immune suppressive effects of stress. It also moisturizes and soothes immune organ membranes.

LEMON PEEL
Place the peel of a lemon and squeeze a little of the flesh juice into a cup of warm water.

PAU D'ARCO TEA
This tea contains an active compound called lapachol, which is antifungal, antiparasitic and antimicrobial. It also helps to maintain the integrity of red blood cells and other immune-supporting organs. If you ever feel that you are coming down with something or feel under the weather, this is the tea for you.

ECHINACEA
Echinacea helps to maintain immunity and clear infections. It is available in tincture, tablet and tea form, best to take in rotation; one week on, one week off.

STRESS-RELATED BACKACHES ON THE RISE

My clinical experience tells me that backaches are on the rise due to stress and poor nutrition. It is worth considering that the spine is a major pathway for the nerves of the body. All emotional, psychological and physical stresses can therefore manifest in the back, especially the lower back – the seat of your kidneys. The kidneys are a purification system for the body. When you are under stress or your body is malnourished from a poor diet, the kidneys have to work overtime and their purifying system may not work as efficiently. Therefore, nutrition can play a vital role in the prevention of backaches.

NUTRITIONAL BACKACHE HELP

► Drink more water, at least 6–8 glasses a day. Dehydration will cause backache even in those who are not normally prone to back afflictions. Water also helps flush out the excess acid particles from the kidneys.

► Avoid red meats, caffeine and, in some cases, dairy from cow's milk (if you have a line down the middle of your tongue, this is an indication that you are unable to digest the large molecules of cow's milk). Sugar, alcohol and processed foods may also aggravate your back.

► Eat more green leafy veggies. Nuts such as walnuts and almonds, seeds and cold-water fish are good food choices too. Add more raw fruits, vegetables and whole grains to your diet.

► Reduce the bad fats in your diet. Bad fats create compounds in the body that contribute to spinal disc degeneration.

► Ensure that you have an adequate supply of magnesium and calcium in the diet (see page 99).

► If you suffer from lower back problems, take the following supplements every day:
  ► Magnesium (1000mg)
  ► Calcium (750mg)
  ► Silica (1–2 tablespoons of liquid silica)
  ► Liquid minerals
  ► Green juice drinks to flush out acids
  ► Boron (3mg) for better uptake of the above nutrients
  ► Aloe vera juice (2 tablespoons) an hour before bed

CHAPTER 5

CLEAN OUT

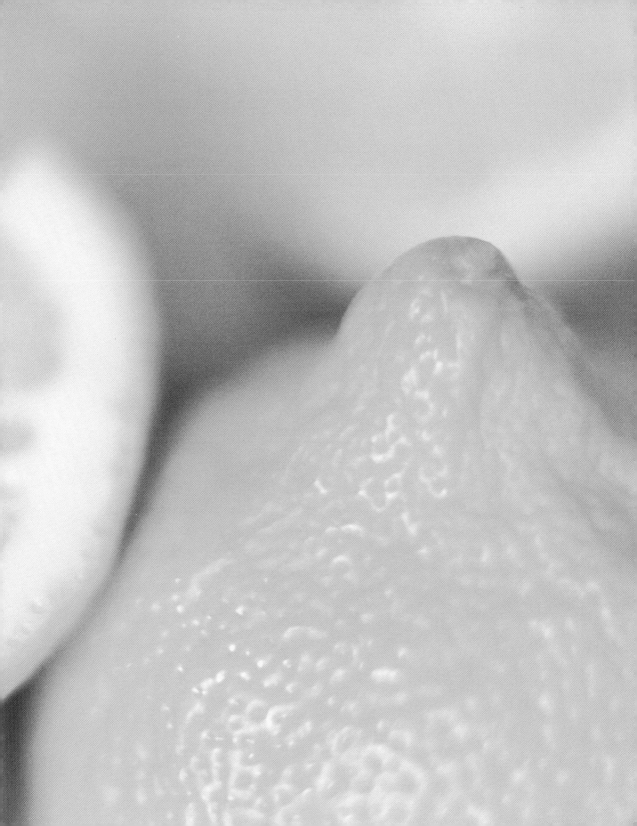

First, I just met a martial arts instructor who went on a regime of only carrot and cucumber juice for thirty days. Simply put, he was exhausted.

Second, a close friend of mine once checked in for a detox at a center in California to, in her own words, "cleanse the arteries of chocolate and ice cream." For three weeks, she could only eat a few teaspoons of alfalfa sprouts and clover sprouts in a whole day. If she was really good, she was permitted a thin slice of watermelon at the end of the week as a reward. When she left the center, she could only think about one thing: eating a big hamburger, and eating it right now. And this was a woman who hadn't eaten red meat for years.

Lastly, a work colleague of mine went on a "mung bean and rice detox fast." This beanpole of a man ate nothing else but mung beans and brown rice for sixty days straight, breakfast, lunch and dinner. He said that the diet made him feel "a bit dizzy, light-headed, like fainting at times" but it would help him to "meet his soul."

Everybody on my TV show *You Are What You Eat* had a colonic to go along with their new food changes. One participant loved the results so much that he went on a course of ten colonics. His first colonic was like a volcanic eruption. So much undigested food particles (putting it politely) that had been trying to escape for years had finally found freedom in one gigantic rush. He lost several pounds that day!

The fact is that a detox of any sort needn't be this dramatic or extreme, nor need it be unpleasant or inconvenient. A detox can be gentle, easy, simple and minimal. And a detox should not be so austere that you would kill for a chocolate bar because you are in such desperation.

Our bodies are automatically detoxing every day anyway. The body has natural physiological detox actions of its own: sweating, urinating and moving bowels for example. But in our modern era of pollutants, heavy metals, computer and cell phone radiations, cigarettes, harsh cleaning solvents, industrial sprays, chemical pesticides, military coordinates, alcohol and more, the human body has become immensely overloaded with various toxicities. Our bodies need a little help every so often.

Patients who have implemented my simple detox tips for everyday life, and then embarked upon my easy Detox Day plan, were able to eradicate all kinds of health problems, including:

- Low sex drive
- Infertility
- Impotency
- PMS
- Indigestion
- Ovarian cysts

- Headaches
- Joint pains
- Bad breath
- Allergies
- Constipation
- Brittle nails

- Skin eruptions
- Poor memory
- Depression
- Insomnia
- Excess weight

And most important, they feel great! In the first part of this chapter, I will give you my six simple tips you can incorporate into your daily routine. This will keep your body relatively toxic-free. Then in the second part, you can follow my Detox Day plan.

WHY DETOX?

The body stores foreign substances and toxins in its fatty deposits. So, in many cases, people may be carrying up to ten or more extra pounds (4.5kg) of unhealthy mucus-harboring toxic waste!

And you wonder why you are so tired, have PMS, digestive disorders, headaches, joint pains, bad breath, allergies, constipation, brittle nails, skin eruptions, poor memory, depression, insomnia, excess weight and so on. It is a toxic world we live in, and you may be living in an increasingly toxic body.

For a time, your body will struggle to protect itself from noxious toxins by trapping them in a ball of mucus or fat so that they are impeded from triggering adverse immune reactions. But this Band-Aid will only last temporarily. Before long, the toxins will seep into the bloodstream and into cell membranes, disturbing metabolic function and causing tissue damage.

If I still haven't convinced you then take the Detox Challenge and see if your body is need of a cleanse.

WHAT IS A TOXIN?

A toxin can be any kind of substance that causes harmful effects to the body, leading to intolerances, allergies and a general feeling of illness. We are surrounded by potential toxins from the water we drink, the food we eat and the air we breathe. The most insidious toxins are actually not seen, invisible, leaving us unaware as to the grave risks. The good news, though, is that the body has a gift of being able to expel toxins quite readily if we have the knowledge, tools and my Plan to rid them.

TAKE THE DETOX CHALLENGE

Answer yes or no to each of the following questions:

Do you live in a city?

Do you work in an office?

Do you use underground transport regularly?

Do you frequently jog, run or walk alongside busy roads with traffic?

Do you regularly use a cell phone?

Do you regularly use a computer?

Do you live near high-voltage power lines, a nuclear or electrical power plant or cell phone tower(s)?

Do you regularly smoke cigarettes or other substances?

Do you frequently use recreational or prescription drugs and medications?

Do you drink alcohol on a daily basis, or binge-drink on the weekends or at other times?

Do you lead a sedentary lifestyle whereby you never exercise?

Do you catch more than three colds, flus and/or viruses in an average year?

Do you have any mercury fillings in your teeth?

Do you drink on a daily basis any of the following: coffee, fizzy drinks, tap water, cows' milk and/or carbonated sodas?

Do you eat on a daily basis any of the following: sugar, sweets, chocolates, white bread, canned foods, frozen foods, microwaved foods, fried foods, meats, cured lunch meats, cookies, cakes?

Do you normally add white sugar or sugar substitutes to tea or coffee?

Do you regularly add salt to your food when cooking, or add salt when the dish arrives?

Is reading food labels for chemicals or preservatives before making selections irrelevant to you?

SCORING

If you answered yes to more than five questions, then you may be a toxic junkie. I suggest you embark upon my Detox Day Plan at your earliest convenience. This weekend perhaps?

If you answered yes to more than ten questions, then you are a toxic dump monster. You are most likely loaded with toxins throughout your organs, cells, blood and body. You might even have bad breath, flatulence and body odor. If not, you'll have it soon enough along with a host of serious ills if you fail to act immediately. Therefore, you must embark upon my Detox Day Plan immediately. And I mean today. I am not giving you a choice here!

The good news is that a detox of any sort need not be unpleasant, undignified or inconvenient. A detox can be gentle, easy, simple and minimal. It certainly shouldn't be so austere that it makes you want to kill for a doughnut because you are in such desperation.

MY SIMPLE EVERYDAY DETOX TIPS

I HAVE FOUND THAT PATIENTS WHO IMPLEMENT MY SIMPLE DETOX TIPS FOR EVERYDAY LIFE, AND THEN EMBARK UPON MY EASY ONE-DAY DETOX, ARE ABLE TO LOSE WEIGHT MUCH MORE EASILY. THEY ARE ALSO ABLE TO ERADICATE ALL KINDS OF HEALTH PROBLEMS INCLUDING: LOW SEX DRIVE, INFERTILITY, IMPOTENCY, PMS, INDIGESTION, MALABSORPTION, OVARIAN CYSTS, HEADACHES, JOINT PAINS, BAD BREATH, ALLERGIES, CONSTIPATION, BRITTLE NAILS, SKIN ERUPTIONS, POOR MEMORY, DEPRESSION, INSOMNIA, EXCESS WEIGHT ... THE LIST GOES ON. MOST IMPORTANT, THE PEOPLE WHO FOLLOW MY DETOX TIPS FEEL GREAT! HERE, I WILL GIVE YOU SIX SIMPLE TIPS THAT YOU CAN INCORPORATE INTO YOUR DAILY ROUTINE TO KEEP YOUR BODY RELATIVELY TOXIN-FREE. I WILL THEN FOLLOW WITH THE ONE-DAY DETOX.

Remember, these tips are not just one-offs; they're meant for everyday life.

Body brushing purges the garbage and toxins from your system. Give it a go and you will feel like a new person.

1 STUDY THE TOP FOODS LIST BELOW

Be sure to keep it handy at all times, because it will show you which are the most detoxifying foods for everyday life and which are the most toxic.

Top Detox Foods

- Fruit and vegetable juices
- Water
- Raw food/sprouts/greens
- Fruits, veggies, whole grains, legumes, seeds

Foods to Avoid

- Sugar
- Fried foods
- Dairy
- Alcohol
- Caffeine

2 BUY AND START USING THE FOLLOWING ITEMS TODAY

- A **juicer** to start making your own vegetable juices. Don't worry about buying the most expensive model – just get whatever you can afford. Once you really get into the juicing, you can look for fancier, quicker models later on.
- A **blender** to start making your own delicious, easy-to-digest smoothies.

3 START SKIN BRUSHING

Buy a skin brush and please make sure you use it. Dry skin brushing speeds up the rate at which toxins are expelled from the body, because it motivates blood cells and lymph tissue, two key physiological detoxification avenues. Skin brushing is not something you do in the bath or shower, but when you are dry. You can bathe afterward but not during the process.

Method:
Smoothly brush the soles of the feet, working your way up the legs, then up the arms and down the back. Brush in long sweeping movements towards your heart, as it increases circulation and improves skin tone and texture. Always brush lightly and gently, and avoid broken skin, thread veins and varicose veins.

4 BREATHE!

The way you breathe can have a dramatic effect on your health – oxygen is a powerful detoxifier. Deep breathing is the key. Most people breathe in a shallow manner, thus depriving the cells, organs and glands of much-needed oxygen. Oxygen literally feeds the blood and cells, as it detoxifies the organs and glands, and is just as important as adequate supplies of water and good-quality food. A lack of it actually starves the brain, nervous system, adrenals, pituitary, kidneys, gall bladder, spleen, liver, diaphragm and colon.

In my breathing method I'll expect you to adopt more full and ample breathing from the lower diaphragm, while filling the entire lungs on a regular daily basis. But in order to get to a point where deep breathing becomes a part of your everyday life, I would like you to practice the following breathing method for just a few minutes each day. Once you master it, you will find it so much easier to incorporate deep breathing into normal life, when you're walking, talking, sitting, working or relaxing.

Method:

- Lie on your back on the floor in a position that is most comfortable for you: For instance, you might want your knees bent and your feet apart. Close your eyes if it helps you to relax.
- Place one hand on your tummy and one hand on your chest. Then breathe deeply. Which moves first: the hand on your chest or the hand on your tummy? If the answer is the hand on your chest, then you are not using your lungs to optimum capacity. You are undoubtedly starving your cells and organs of oxygen.
- Now slowly breathe in through the nose. Count to 10 if it helps you to focus.
- Make an *oooh* sound slowly through your lips. Then blow out any remaining air as gently and slowly as possible, simultaneously applying light pressure to your lower abdomen to help expel all stale air.
- Slowly inhale through your nostrils, keeping one hand on your stomach just above your belly button. Visualize your breath literally expanding throughout the lungs, ribs and sides (middle and upper segments of the back). It's like putting air into a balloon. When you inhale, it fills with air. This air expands to your sides, ribs and back. When you exhale, the balloon deflates.
- When you breathe out, feel the ribs move down and your tension melting away as the tummy and upper body deflate. Repeat the *oooh* sound, and gently blow out air, completely emptying your lungs. Once you become more experienced, you may not need to make this sound.

You don't need to over-breathe while doing this. It's meant to be a slow, gentle, calming, meditative exercise. Use visualization (to see or) to think about the slow movements of the air, and, most importantly, feel calmness, tranquillity and serenity as you do it.

5 EXERCISE DAILY

In order to properly detox the body, exercise is essential. I am not suggesting you have to embark upon a vigorous body-building plan that takes you to the local gym each day. I am talking about simple, gentle movement – the type that will keep your body nimble, supple and young! Some stretching, walking, step-climbing, mini-trampolining, dancing, salsa, disco, swimming, bicycling, aerobics, Pilates, even tai chi or karate if you can find it in your neighborhood, or any other moderate fun movements would be excellent on a regular basis. Anything that makes you break into a sweat is even better.

6 DRINK WATER

Regularly drinking still water – not from the tap unless it is filtered – is one of the most efficient detoxifying fluids we can give ourselves each day. I recommend 6–8 glasses of water a day.

DR. GILLIAN'S DETOX DAY

FOR THE DETOXIFICATION PROCESS TO WORK PROPERLY, YOU SHOULD NOT STARVE YOURSELF. YOU WILL SIMPLY GIVE YOUR ORGANS A HOLIDAY FROM WHAT YOU NORMALLY EAT. YOU WILL CUT OUT THE NAUGHTY FOODS, ADD LOTS OF GOOD FOODS THAT CLEANSE YOUR ORGANS AND FACILITATE THE EXPULSION OF TOXINS FROM YOUR BODY. AND AS A RESULT YOU WILL BRIM WITH VITALITY AND ENERGY.

THE NAUGHTY FOODS: DANGER ... STAY AWAY!

On your Detox Day, say goodbye completely to foods that destroy your cells, drain your energies, are difficult to digest and sap your vitality. Here is a list of Naughties. And if you can stay away from the Naughties for longer, then more power to you! It will do you the world of good and make your path to a slimmer, healthier you even easier.

AVOID THE FOLLOWING:

- ► Coffee
- ► Seafood
- ► Sugar
- ► Tea
- ► Milk
- ► Salt and pepper
- ► Cigarettes
- ► Eggs
- ► Carbonated beverages
- ► Alcohol
- ► Cheese
- ► Fried foods
- ► Red meat
- ► Cooking oil
- ► Commercial mayonnaise
- ► Poultry
- ► Bread
- ► Mustard
- ► Fish
- ► Medications (unless you have a preexisting condition that requires them)

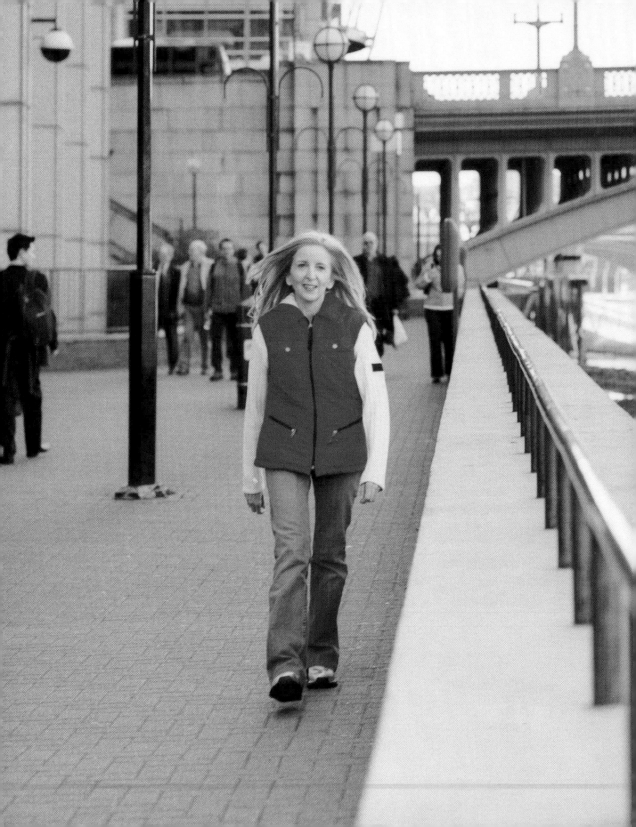

EXERCISE

The most important thing is that you do something that's fun on your Detox Day. You don't need a partner for this. Simply turn on the radio, find a tune you like and start dancing. It's great fun, moves your blood and circulatory system, tones your bod and lifts your spirits. And if you have children at home, they too will love to dance with you. You can do it together with anyone or just yourself, have fun and rejuvenate all your bodies at the same time.

Keep dancing for thirty to forty-five minutes if you want a decent aerobic workout. I tell my patients who work at sitting jobs to get up every hour on the hour and dance their brains out for five minutes. But on your Detox Day, feel free to do whatever feels right for you without overdoing it. By flexing, moving, stretching and relaxing the muscles, the lymph fluid effectively pulls out toxins. Sweating does the same.

THE FOLLOWING SUPPLEMENTS SHOULD BE TAKEN DURING YOUR DETOX DAY, AS THEY WILL ASSIST CLEANSING OF THE LIVER, BOWELS AND CELLS WHILE SUPPORTING YOUR OVERALL CONSTITUTION STRENGTH:

1 GREEN SUPERFOODS

You need to make sure that you have 2 generous teaspoons of a green superfood on your Detox Day. Choose any one or more of the following:

- ► Wild blue-green algae
- ► Spirulina
- ► Chlorella
- ► Wheatgrass
- ► Barley grass
- ► Dr. Gillian McKeith's Living Food Energy Powder

2 DIGESTIVE ENZYMES

Take as instructed or with any warm meals/drinks.

3 LINSEEDS OR FLAX OIL

1 tablespoon of either daily.

4 MILK THISTLE

Take milk thistle or alpha lipoic acid to support your detox organs (2 capsules daily) (If you wish, open the capsule contents and pour into one of your juices in the middle of day.) To check if you need milk thistle or alpha lipoic acid supplements take a look at the symptoms in the box opposite. If you tick even just one, then you will need to take either milk thistle or alpha lipoic acid during your detox – and for two weeks afterward.

5 ACIDOPHILUS

If you opt for an enema or colonic hydrotherapy, you will need acidophilus supplements.

6 SPROUTS

Learn how to grow your own grasses and sprouts. See page 213 to learn how, or buy them ready sprouted.

7 DR. GILLIAN McKEITH'S 24-HOUR DETOX

For those who desire a good inside clean-out but may not want a colonic.

DO YOU NEED MILK THISTLE?

Nausea	Anger	Insomnia
Headaches	Post-partum depression	Dizziness
Digestive upset	Irritability	Tinnitus
Hemorrhoids	Aggressive	Hot palms
Bruising	Tense	Hot soles
Moody	Splitting nails	Painful eyes
Depression	Red eyes	Red face
Blurry vision	Tenderness under right rib	Amalgam fillings
Quivering tongue (tongue shakes a bit when you stick it out)		

DR. GILLIAN'S DETOX DAY: STEP-BY-STEP

ON RISING
(Times may be modified to your personal lifestyle):

7:00AM WARM LEMON WATER
Squeeze some fresh lemon into warm water as desired. Warm water with lemon allows a gentle start to the day, as it goes straight through to the bowels, helping to expel fecal matter from the day before. (Cold water, first thing in the morning, shocks and stops at the tummy, thus creating gas or bloating.)

7:30AM LINSEED
Choose from:
▶ Place 2 heaped teaspoons of organic linseeds in a large glass of filtered water.
▶ Soak 1 tablespoon of linseeds in a cup of boiling water the night before. Drink *only* the liquid in the morning.

8:00AM BREAKFAST
Choose from:
▶ Fruit. Your breakfast fruit should be served at room temperature. Eat enough so that you are not hungry and chew it really well. Avoid oranges or orange juice as they are too acidic. If you opt for grapes, don't mix them with anything else. Choose from: apples, pears, papayas, pineapples, cherries, peaches, plums, watermelons, apricots, berries.
▶ Miso soup
▶ Vegetable juice, made up of: 1 cucumber, 1/4 piece of root ginger (peeled), 4 celery stalks, 100g (4oz) alfalfa sprouts, 3 sprigs parsley, and 1 carrot (peeled).

9:30AM TEA BREAK: DRINK A CUP OR TWO OF HERBAL TEA

During this Detox Day, we will take several tea breaks. After all, what would we do without our tea breaks? So this day is no different. I have built in a number of them for your sipping pleasure. Nutritionally speaking, though, my tea breaks will be nourishing, healing and will enhance the detox. You will need to choose from the list of teas that I tell you. You cannot drink your regular caffeine-laden black tea, but you can drink: nettle, dandelion, camomile, sage or echinacea teas.

10:00AM FRUIT JUICE BREAK

Choose seasonal fruit, freshly squeezed or pressed with your juicer – see overleaf for some ideas. If it's winter and/or you feel chilly, then add some boiling hot water to the juice. If you are getting rather hungry mid-morning, then please make more juices for yourself.

If one or more of the following applies to you, please warm your fruit either by gentle steaming or placing fruit in a pan of warm water (you are not boiling the fruit, simply warming it):

▸ It is wintertime and/or you do not live in a warm climate.
▸ You feel cold or have poor circulation.
▸ You have a weak spleen. (You can easily tell this by looking at your tongue in a mirror. See page 34 for tongue signs of a weak spleen.)

WARM APPLE DELIGHT

6 apples
2 pears

▸ Peel, core and chop the fruit. Steam lightly and blend.
Take 1 digestive enzyme capsule with this warmed fruit delicacy.
Simply open up the capsule and pour the contents into the blend.

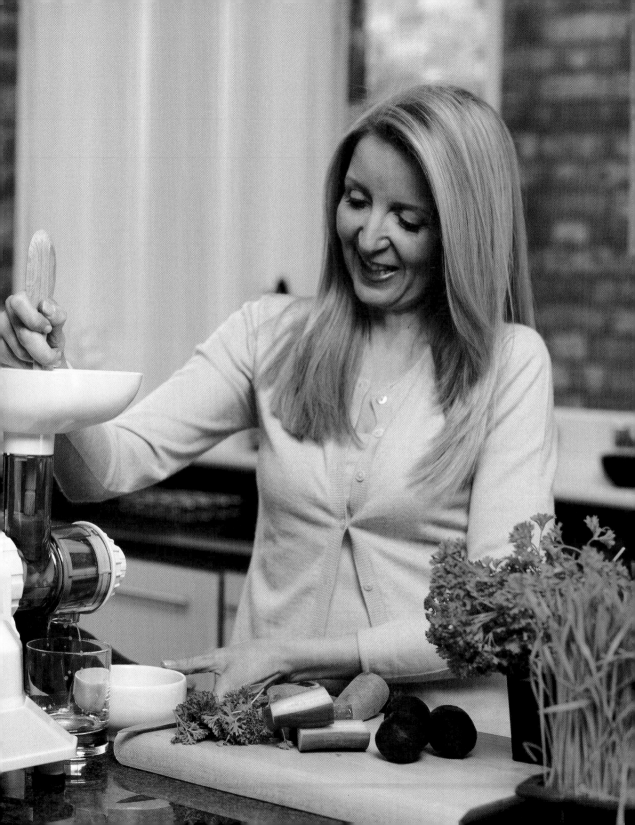

JUICING IDEAS

All fruits and vegetables should be peeled and cored before juicing.
Ginger root should be peeled and grated.

SPROUT SURPRISE
1 apple, 175g (6oz) alfalfa sprouts or clover sprouts,
6 fresh mint leaves, 3 carrots

LEMON ESSENCE
8 carrots, 1 apple, juice of 1 lemon, 2.5cm (1 inch) slice ginger root

PAPAYA PARADE
2 firm papayas, 2 pears, ½ teaspoon grated ginger root

GRAPES GALORE
20 green grapes, 10 strawberries, 1 apple, 2 sprigs fresh mint

GINGER ENLIVENER
2 apples, 2 pears, small piece of ginger root
This is a terrific breakfast enlivener that will perk up your whole system,
providing a wake-up call for the taste buds too.

BERRY BLITZ
1 pint of your favorite berries or even mixed berries (strawberries,
blackberries, gooseberries, raspberries), 2 peaches, 1 apple

PINEAPPLE PICK-ME-UP
Juice of 1 pineapple

12:30PM LUNCH

You've made it so far. And I'll bet you're doing just fine.
Now here's lunch.
Choose from one of the following:

- Raw salad with sprouts
- Raw Mint Cucumber Soup
- Raw sauerkraut
- Grain such as millet, quinoa, rice, amaranth
  After cooking the grain (see page 66), add one or more of the following raw herbs to mix with it: dill, chives, chervil, or dandelion leaves. Serve with a side dish of broccoli, cauliflower, cabbage, cucumber, dark green lettuce leaves, celery or Brussels sprouts.

DR. GILLIAN'S RAW MINT CUCUMBER SOUP

Juice of 3 cucumbers and 2 celery sticks
1 cucumber, chopped
¼ cup fresh chopped mint leaves
¼ cup fresh chopped parsley
¼ leek, finely chopped

Put all ingredients in a food processor or blender and blend until smooth.

2:00PM HERBAL TEA BREAK

2:30PM DR. MCKEITH'S VEGGIE DETOX JUICE
Choose from the following freshly made juices using your juicer:

COOL CARROTMANIA
This is delightful and very nourishing to the liver.
6 carrots, 2 celery stalks and 1 apple.
(Try a version without apple too.)

BEETROOT BLAST
1/2 beetroot, 2 carrots, 1 celery stalk, 1/2 a small cucumber

COOL CUCUMBER
2 whole cucumbers, 1/4–1/2 beetroot, a dill sprig

CUCUMBER MEDLEY
2 cucumbers, 4 celery stalks, 1/4 of a piece of root ginger (optional),
sprig of basil or coriander
This is my favorite.

GREENS TO GO
A handful of parsley, 1 kale leaf, 5 carrots and a tiny piece of root ginger

CELERY ENERGY
2 celery stalks, a handful of parsley, 1 garlic clove, 5 carrots and 100g
(4oz) alfalfa sprouts (optional but great if you do)

3:00PM HERBAL TEA BREAK

3:30PM IT'S SNACK TIME!
Snack on sunflower seeds, pumpkin seeds and/or raw sauerkraut.

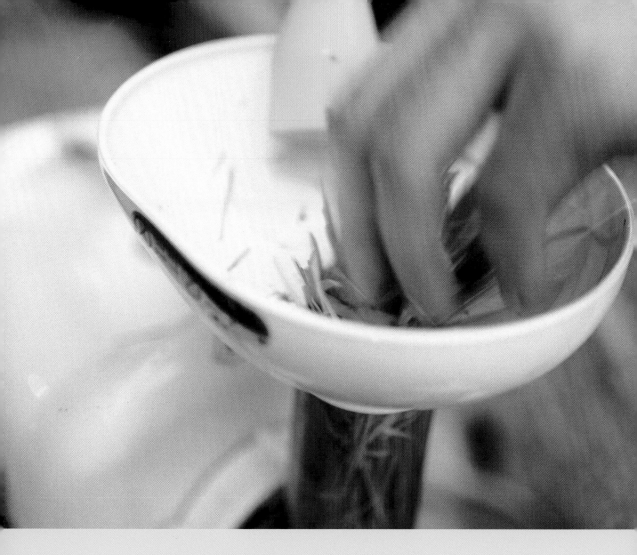

4:00 PM DR. GILLIAN'S DELECTABLE VEGGIE SMOOTHIE

6 carrots (with tops if possible)
1 soft avocado
10 basil leaves
1 apple
1 lemon slice

Juice the carrots and apple through a juicer. Add to the other ingredients and blend in a blender or food processor. Squeeze a dash of lemon into the drink.

5:30PM DINNER

You are almost finished for the day. You can now eat a hearty raw salad with a handful of raw sprouts. Plus, add a small amount of grain if feeling really hungry.

6:30PM POTASSIUM BROTH BREAK

You are doing very well. Keep it up.

PLEASE DON'T FRET!

If it's too much effort or you really cannot be bothered with the Potassium Broth thing, then please don't worry about it. Instead, get over to your local health food store, and buy some miso soup packs. All you have to do is add boiling water and drink. Really easy!

WHAT'S THIS WITH THE POTASSIUM BROTH?

Potassium Broth infuses a cocktail of minerals and vitamins – especially potassium for electrolyte balance – into the body's organs, glands and tissues. Mineral imbalance is a catalyst for decreased organ function. I want to keep up your mineral profile while infusing you with vitamins too.

POTASSIUM BROTH

(Always wash all produce thoroughly, but no need to peel the skins if you are going organic.)

Ingredients

2 large potatoes
2 carrots
1 cup red beets (optional)
4 celery stalks with leaves
1 cup parsley
1 cup turnips
A pinch of cayenne, to taste

Use stainless steel utensils and pots. Fill a large saucepan with approximately 1.8L (3½ pints) of water. Slice the vegetables directly into water – never leave your veggies sitting around waiting for ages. Bring to the boil, then reduce the heat. Cover and cook on a low temperature (a very light simmer) for 2 hours or so. Strain the vegetables and drink **only** the broth.

7:30PM WARM WATER WITH LEMON BREAK

Just squeeze fresh lemon into a teacup with warm or hot water and drink.

8:15PM DRY SKIN BRUSH

(See page 132.)

8:30PM YOUR REWARD: A MINERAL BATH

You made it this far; you deserve an accolade. An amazing bath
is your reward. This is not just for women, by the way. Men will also
enjoy this soothing, mineral-rich bath. Once the bath is filled with
water, add the following (all available from health food stores):
2 teaspoons flax oil
some liquid minerals
1 teaspoon liquid silica
2 teaspoons aloe vera
3 or 4 drops each of the essential oils of frankincense and myrrh
This will probably be the most expensive bathwater you've ever had
to let drain away! But be aware that the skin is the largest and most
absorbent organ we have. And so all of these nutrients, in the bathwater,
will be absorbed most efficiently through your pores and other obvious
openings.

9:00PM THOSE LATE-NIGHT MUNCHIES

Munch on lettuce and celery stalks before bedtime. (Celery is loaded
with the mineral magnesium, one of the most calming nutrients.)
Get to bed early (between 9:30pm and 10:30pm) if you can.

Just one or more of the following herbal and plant leaves can add a real zip to your juices. You can either put them through the juicer, or mix the leaves and juice together through a blender.

- Basil
- Chives
- Coriander
- Dill

- Fennel
- Fenugreek
- Garlic
- Ginger

- Lemongrass
- Spearmint

Sprouted seeds, such as fenugreek and radish, can also be added to your juices to spice things up and further warm you up.

WHAT IF I'M HUNGRY?

If you experience hunger attacks, you can drink more herbal teas, miso broth or juice. Warm soup is fine if you feel cold or if it's chilly outside. Plenty of liquid is important – aim for 2 quarts per day (can be a combination of juices and plain water). The problem is that many people don't drink enough liquid needed to flush out accumulated toxins. In addition, the juices and herbal teas will act like natural diuretics, lessening the possibility of water retention.

Finally, I tell all my patients that there's no need to be a slave to the juice. If you need to, you can eat some solid fruit and/or vegetables, even salad and seeds. If you absolutely must, amaranth, millet or quinoa are good grains to include. It may take some time before your body is ready to accept a full day of juicing. Don't force it before it is ready; listen to your gut feeling.

THE HEALING CRISIS

During or after a detox, some people experience what is referred to as a healing crisis. This means that the elimination or detoxification was so efficient or so powerful that they can feel unwell for a few days or few hours during or afterward. My patients are usually spared because of the gentle and nutritionally balanced manner in which I conduct the detox. If anything, you will probably feel energized, clearheaded, rejuvenated and revitalized. But there is always a chance that you may still have an adverse feeling from such deep elimination. You may experience headaches, joint pains, skin eruptions, and more. Don't be alarmed by these symptoms – you can stop the detox whenever you like and go back to gradually incorporating the detox principles in your everyday diet.

EMOTIONAL REACTIONS

Another form of healing crisis is the emotional crisis which some people might experience when going through a deep detox. Don't be surprised if you feel weepy or emotional when you start detoxing – you may find that years of pent-up tensions may be processed and released.

THE DETOX MASSAGE

Take five minutes in the morning and evening of your Detox Day to rub your liver region. Simply lie flat on your back and gently massage the liver using your fingertips. This will further spur the detoxification process, and although it may not sound like it at first, it can feel really nice too!

Method:
You will find your liver at the base of your right ribcage. Simply place your hand at the bottom of the set of ribs on your right side. Move your fingers in a clockwise direction around the liver for approximately five minutes. Do not dig into your liver with your nails; use your fingertips, take it slowly and gently. You will be helping to stimulate the liver-cleansing action and the processing of body toxins.

GOING ALL THE WAY TO GET IT OUT

Some people may prefer to extend their detox to two, three and even four days. This is okay if you feel ready and if you have previously experimented with the Detox Day on another occasion. There is no right or wrong here. It's about educating yourself with proper information and listening to your feelings.

DIG DEEPER : CLEAN OUT THE DIRTY SINK

If you never cleaned your sink, think what it would look like. Your Detox Day is like a spring clean, but you can dig deeper too with the help of enemas and colonics. You can either buy an enema kit from a pharmacy (instructions are supplied) or you can treat yourself to a colonic hydrotherapy treatment. Either way, it's best if you do the enema or colonic on the day of your cleanse, in the evening perhaps. If you can spare the time, have a treatment one to two days before your Detox Day in addition to the Detox Day itself. It's not something you have to do but it can be very helpful, increasing the level of cleansing in one swoop so to speak. Think about it and go with it if it feels right for you.

THE COLON: YOUR CRITICAL ORGAN

The colon, large intestine or bowel is situated in the abdominal region and forms the last part of the digestive tract. An extremely important organ in its own right, it carries out a number of vital functions including the completion of the digestive process involving absorption of water, assimilation of minerals, as well as the synthesis of vitamins.

The colon is a major part of the excretory system, and is responsible for eliminating food and other body wastes, as well as protecting us from infection and disease. In a normally functioning colon, all this is achieved with the help of billions of friendly bacteria which inhabit the colon and make up some 70 percent of the dry weight of our fecal waste.

However, the delicate balance of this internal ecosystem can very easily be disturbed by a number of factors including stress, pollution, electromagnetic influences, poor food and drink choices, medications, smoking and exposure to toxic substances. The worse your colon is, the quicker you will age. Your own internal filth could be slowly poisoning you.

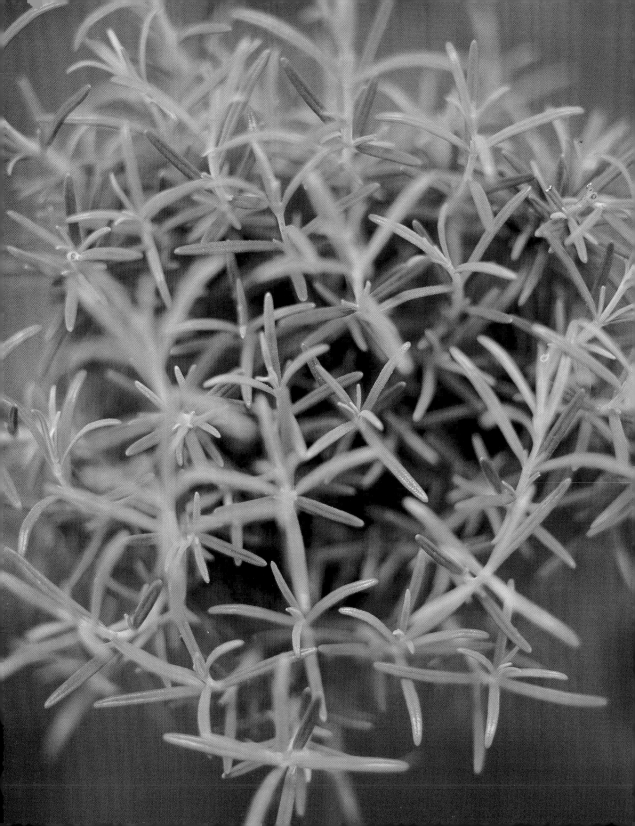

COLONIC HYDROTHERAPY

I often describe colonic hydrotherapy as an enema, except that it's forty times more powerful in terms of cleaning out the colon. The colonic hydrotherapy procedure gently sends warm, sterile water into your lower bowel and colon to assist in cleansing years of excess mucus, gas, fecal matter, pollutants, medication and toxic substances.

Whether you opt for this or an enema, make sure you take some beneficial bacteria afterward. You can buy beneficial bacteria supplements in any health food store. They often have different names – look for the words "probiotics," "acidophilus" or "beneficial bacteria" – and simply ask for help if you're not completely sure. The supplements come in either powder or capsule form. If you have capsules, open up two, pour the contents into a little water and sip slowly.

According to the International Colonic Association, colonic hydrotherapy is often beneficial for weight loss, constipation, hemorrhoids, colitis, yeast infections, diarrhea and other conditions, and may even help to prevent cancer of the colon. The treatments often result in increased energy, advanced mental clarity, clearer skin, improved circulation, enhanced immunity and proper weight control for the patient. The procedure itself will take approximately forty-five minutes. You lie down on a comfortable table for the treatment. A tube is then slightly inserted into your anus. This does not hurt, nor is it painful; you might feel a mild pressure, but nothing else. Just don't get hung up on it! The benefits are worth it.

Depending on the therapist, abdominal massage may be administered to aid in the movement of trapped gas pockets and waste matter. You can usually see what is coming out. (Psychologically speaking, this can be good for many people.) At my clinic in London, it is not unusual to view whole pieces of broccoli or other food items sailing through the colonic tube – obviously not properly chewed. Remember, your colon does not have teeth! The feeling of a colonic is akin to the feeling you have when you produce a bowel movement. The key is to relax, let go and embrace the cleaning out of your insides.

Colonics are the perfect complement to my Detox Day, but I am quite happy if you don't want to opt for one. They are not everybody's cup of tea. The most important thing is to at least implement the other six simple detox tips at the beginning of this chapter, and please embark upon my Detox Day every so often, say once every other month or so. It's all so simple and easy to do, and the health benefits will be immense.

For colonic cowards: If you don't fancy a colonic, then get my Dr. Gillian McKeith 24-Hour Detox. It's the only detox that will clean you out in a day. (www.drgillianmckeith.com)

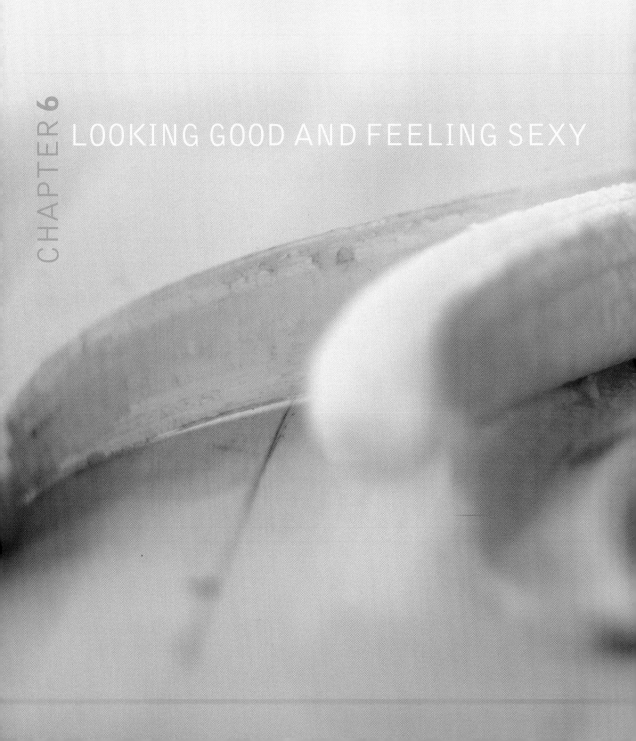

CHAPTER 6

LOOKING GOOD AND FEELING SEXY

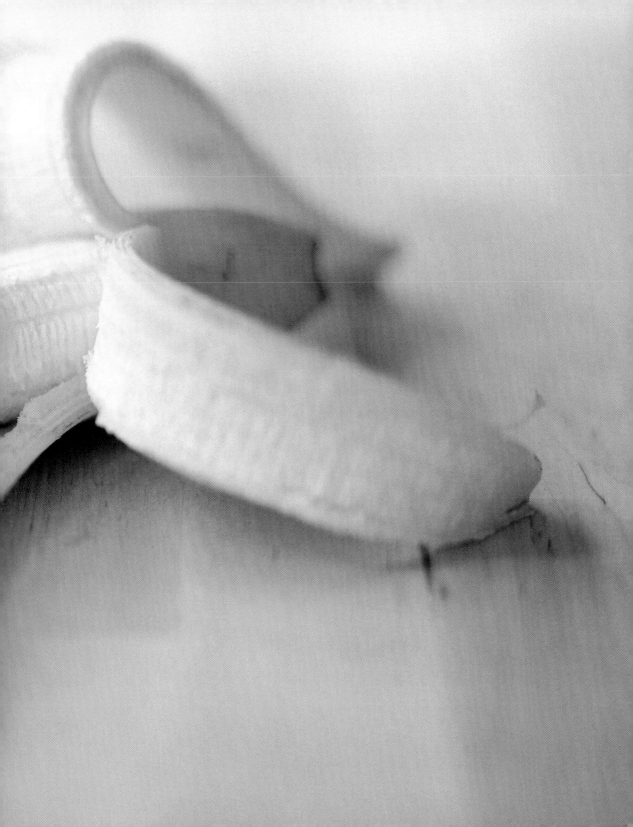

When I was in my early twenties I was embarrassed by the way I looked – and especially about my forehead, which was covered in pimples. So one day I took a pair of scissors to my hair and cut this hideous fringe, which I did not suit, to cover the blemishes. That way no one would have to see them, not even me. My new silly-looking fringe could cover up the pimples! I was too embarrassed to have a professional hairdresser style the front, as I didn't want anyone to even notice me, and I can remember avoiding mirrors like the plague. If a room had a mirror, I would stay away. If I couldn't stay away from the room – a bathroom with a mirror, say – I would actually dim the lights. I simply didn't want to have to look at myself in a mirror for fear of what I'd see.

But in those days, living away from home, I ate a lot of what I now call goo and gloo foods (cheese, milk, fatty meats, pastries, junk food, sugar, chocolate) plus a little too much alcohol, on occasion, without understanding the consequences. Foods like this encourage the formation of mucus around the colon, and clog the blood-cleansing capability of organs with the result that blood cannot be purified properly. And when the organs and the blood are overburdened, toxins are often excreted in the skin. So, with my pimples, I looked like what I was made up of. I was the quintessential example of being You Are What You Eat – I was eating terribly and I looked even worse!

Years later, when I finally stopped eating the wrong foods, the pimples cleared up. I grew out my fringe. And the world and I could view my lovely forehead. I have discovered that the right foods produce creamier skin, thicker hair and stronger nails even though I am older in age.

SKIN CARE

Did you know that skin is the largest organ in your body? It accounts for approximately 16 percent of your total body weight and, besides protecting delicate internal structures, assists the colon, lungs and kidneys in the elimination of toxic waste. It also helps to regulate your body's thermostat by increasing sweat when you get too hot or producing goose pimples when the temperature falls.

Many factors affect the health of your skin, including heredity, age, climate, pollution, diet, stress levels and fluctuations in hormones. However, changes in your complexion are usually swayed by two major factors: (a) how well your internal eliminatory organs are working, (b) whether or not your body is lacking in vitamins and minerals. And both these factors, in turn, influence each other.

Every day in my clinical practice, I see many people who arrive for the first time looking haggard with dry dead skin, pimples, strawlike hair and broken nails. Sure enough, months later, these same patients return looking revived, with beautiful skin, lustrous silky hair, strong long nails. And if you follow my plan I hope you will see such amazing results too.

TEN GOLDEN TIPS FOR HEALTHY SKIN

1 Drink plenty of clean filtered water – at least 6–8 glasses every day, though you might need more during hot weather and on days that you exercise. Adequate water is essential for keeping your skin hydrated and for eliminating toxins through the kidneys and colon.

2 Include lots of fiber in your diet. It keeps your intestinal tract regular, and enhances the elimination of waste products from your body. Some people with skin problems suffer from constipation because they fail to feed themselves with good sources of fiber (see page 105 for a great way to resolve constipation).

3 Make sure your diet contains plenty of antioxidants (which help slow down cellular aging). Fresh fruits and vegetables are the best sources of natural plant antioxidants.

4 Food combine. By eating protein and carbohydrates at separate meals, you'll prevent unnecessary fermentation in the colon and increase nutrient absorption into the blood. See my food-combining program on page 78 in Chapter 3.

5 While bad fats are detrimental to your body, essential fatty acids (good fats) are vital for healthy skin. You can obtain these from whole grains, seeds, nuts, soybeans, dark leafy green vegetables, cold-pressed oils (especially flax, pumpkin, sunflower, sesame and safflower) and oily fish such as sardines, mackerel and wild (not farmed) salmon.

6 On rising, start your day with an early-morning mini-cleanse. This means that you should drink a glass of warm water. Follow this with a mug of nettle tea or hot water with a squeeze of fresh lemon.

7 Avoid excessive amounts of caffeine or alcohol, all of which drain moisture from your body.

8 Cut down on table salt. Excess sodium in the system leads to skin puffiness and swelling. Try celery seeds, sea vegetables, salt-free soy sauce or many of the natural salt-free substitutes. Also avoid strongly spiced dishes where possible.

9 Reduce foods that clog: The worst offenders are red meat, dairy, refined foods, fried foods and foods that contain hydrogenated oils or fats.

10 Externally apply honey three times a week to your face (or any other part of your skin). Leave the honey on the skin approximately 30 minutes. Rinse off honey with warm water (preferably in the shower or bath). You will be amazed by the wonderful results of this simple trick. It will leave your skin soft, supple, young and nourished.

ANTI-ACNE PLAN

Although acne most frequently occurs in teenage years, it can be commonly seen in adults too. It is often due to hormonal imbalances which stimulate the sebaceous glands to increase oil output. But acne can also be due to poor dietary choices. If traces of sebum become trapped inside skin pores, tissues can attract bacteria, resulting in inflammation and blemishes.

Acne is aggravated by poor internal elimination and a high fat and/or refined food diet. Drink plenty of fresh vegetable juices throughout the day: in particular carrot, lettuce, nettle, watercress, celery and dandelion. Also include vegetables and whole grains at both lunchtime and evening meals, particularly green leafy vegetables, carrots, onions, garlic, brown rice, millet and live sprouts.

NUTRITIONAL SUPPLEMENTS

The nutrients I have used most successfully with acne in clinical practice are:
- beta-carotene (25,000iu)
- vitamin A (10,000 iu)
- vitamin B complex (50–100mg)
- pantothenic acid (25mg, four times a day)
- vitamin B6 (50mg)
- propolis (500mg)
- zinc (50mg)
- borage oil capsules daily
- vitamin C (1000mg twice a day)
- Acidophilus with bifidus (friendly bacteria) to promote colon health and elimination of toxins

HERBS

Herbs that are beneficial include echinacea, dandelion, yellow dock, burdock root and red clover; all are powerful internal cleansers. These herbs also support specific organs which synergistically work on the skin.

OTHER TREATMENTS

As an alternative or as a complement to the herbs, try the homeopathic remedy Sulfur 6c. For an external treatment, try bathing the skin with a combination of tea tree oil and camomile (two drops of each in a bowl of water) for a soothing, antibacterial wash.

ANTI-ECZEMA PLAN

Eczema is a form of dermatitis (inflammation of the skin), characterized by flakiness and itching. Associated with sensitivities to both things in your environment or the foods that you eat and are exacerbated by stress, eczema often manifests itself for the first time in new mothers.

Besides cutting out nasty foods in your diet (see Chapter 3, page 74), it would be a good idea to keep a food diary, in case you find a link between your food intake and an eczema outbreak. At different times of stress in life it's quite possible that you may become more sensitive to certain foods that previously caused you no bother. Keep an eye on synthetic allergenic substances such as detergents, solvents, building materials and paints as well.

NUTRITIONAL SUPPLEMENTS

- ► Vitamin B complex (50mg, twice a day)
- ► Vitamin E (400iu, twice a day)
- ► Biotin (100mcg, twice a day)
- ► Zinc (50mg a day)
- ► Plus a source of essential fatty acids (EFAs) such as flax, borage or evening primrose oil

Skin outbreaks are sometimes caused by faulty fat metabolism. High sources of omega-3 and GLA (gamma-linoleic acid, also known as evening primrose oil) are needed in this case. Rotate the EFAs. So, when you've used up the contents of one bottle, switch to a different fatty acid oil. For example, you might take flax oil capsules for one month, and then change to evening primrose oil or borage oil capsules the next month.

OTHER TREATMENTS

Include the homeopathic remedy Graphites 6c where the eczema affects hands and behind the ears; Sulfur 6c where the skin is red, rough and dry and made worse by heat and washing; or Rhus tox 6c where blisters itch more at night but skin feels better with warmth. The topical application of vitamin E and evening primrose oil relieves irritation and promotes the healing process. Calendula cream might also be applied.

ANTI–STRETCH MARK PLAN

More than 80 percent of women get stretch marks at some point in their lives, either from pregnancy or weight gain/loss, and often due to lowered levels of zinc. And men can get them too, usually from rapid weight loss. Stretch marks can fade over time. What starts out as reddish streaks on the skin of the abdomen, breasts, thighs or buttocks, eventually turns into silvery-white thin scars that will never entirely disappear. Many overweight individuals whose skin is well stretched lose weight without any signs of stretch marks. Nutritional and hereditary factors play key roles. To correct zinc deficiency, see the following list of supplements, eat foods high in zinc and take the superfood wild blue-green algae.

NUTRITIONAL SUPPLEMENTS

- ► Vitamin B5 (pantothenic acid) (300mg daily)
- ► Vitamin C with bioflavonoids (1000mg daily)
- ► Vitamin E (600iu daily)
- ► Zinc (at least 15–30mg daily)
- ► Vitamins B5 and C are generally good for the health of the skin.

OTHER TREATMENTS

Certain homeopathic tissue cells salts such as Calc.fluor and Silica help keep cell tissues firm, strong, and elastic. Exercise, in the form of vigorous walking, dancing, swimming and stretching, may also help stretch marks to recede.

DR. McKEITH'S INCREDIBLE EDIBLE ANTI–STRETCH MARK CREAM

Ingredients

½ avocado (soft, ripened)
6 capsules vitamin E
4 capsules vitamin A
2 tablespoons olive oil
2 tablespoons aloe vera gel
5 drops liquid zinc or
2 capsules 50mg zinc powder
½ teaspoon blue-green algae powder (optional)
1 teaspoon silica liquid (optional)

Method

Mash a soft ripe avocado until it forms a creamy paste. Open the capsules of vitamins E and A, and pour the contents of these vitamins into the avocado cream. Add all the other ingredients and mix into the paste. Mix well together. Rub the cream into all relevant areas. Allow the skin to absorb cream for thirty minutes each day. It won't get rid of stretches that are already there, although it may help to lessen their appearance. It also has an incredible softening and nourishing effect on the skin. Your skin will have access to the nutrients it needs to help lessen the future appearance of stretch marks.

Note: Add lemon juice to preserve the cream.

ANTI-VARICOSE VEINS PLAN

Varicose veins are weak or broken spots in surface blood vessels that most commonly occur in the rectum, anus (hemorrhoids) or legs. Besides being unattractive, they might be accompanied by a dull ache, and in more severe cases leg sores may even develop.

There are several factors that are associated with the development of varicose veins, including: prolonged standing or sitting, lack of exercise, obesity, pregnancy and poor food choices. Research also suggests that varicosities run in the family. If your mother or grandfather, for example, had a tendency to the problem, then you may be susceptible as well. By being aware of the possibility, you can take the following necessary steps to avoid or reduce their incidence.

It's interesting to note that in countries where the diet is rich in natural unprocessed foods, varicose veins are virtually unheard of. This is partly due to the high quantities of fiber present in such a regimen and also to the abundance of antioxidant-rich plant foods, which help keep tissues strong and healthy. Avoid eating processed foods. Foods that have an expansive or tiring effect on the cells, such as dairy, sugar, alcohol, conventional tea and coffee, should also be avoided.

AROMATHERAPY VEIN MASSAGE

Add 5 drops of lavender oil and 5 drops of cypress oil to 20ml of carrier oil such as sweet almond or grapeseed. Gently massage into the legs, massaging toward the heart.

NUTRITIONAL SUPPLEMENTS

Rotate the following. You should not take them all at once:

► Vitamin C with bioflavonoids (1000mg twice a day)
► Rutin (500mg twice a day)
► Vitamin E (400iu once a day)
► Vitamin B complex (50mg once a day)
► Coenzyme Q10 (100mg once a day)
► Lecithin 1 (19g twice a day)
► Antioxidant formula (see dosage instructions on package)
► Bilberry herbs (500g, three times a day)

HERBS

► Drink 1 cup of nettle in the morning and 1 cup of horsetail in late afternoon or evening.
► To help ease varicose discomfort, a compress infused with horse chestnut herb can be placed over the affected areas. To prepare the compress mix half a teaspoon of horse chestnut powder with 2 cups of water and use it to soak a sterile cotton cloth.
► Witch hazel herb is another remedy that can also be applied; a natural astringent, it tightens tissues and reduces pain.

OTHER TREATMENTS

Try the homeopathic remedy Hamamelis 30c (1 tablet daily for up to seven days).

*To improve the skin's job of getting
rid of internal garbage (over one pound
of waste products are excreted through
the skin every day), you can help it
in its task by regular body brushing.
To skin brush effectively, you need
a small, firm natural bristle brush.
Brushing is best undertaken just before
you bath or shower on a dry body.
Method: Start at the soles of the feet
and work your way up the legs in long,
brisk strokes; then up the arms and
down the back. Always brush
upward toward the chest and
avoid sensitive spots such as moles,
warts and broken veins. Never
use the brush on your face.*

HAIR AND NAILS

JUST LIKE THE SKIN, THE CONDITION OF YOUR HAIR AND NAILS IS A REVEALING INDICATOR OF YOUR GENERAL WELL-BEING. DIET PLAYS A GREAT PART IN THE HEALTH OF HAIR AND NAILS.

HEALTHY HAIR

As hair is comprised largely of keratin protein, then ample protein levels must be guaranteed. This can be obtained by eating beans, seeds, grains, tofu sprouts and fish. Minerals are also required for hair maintenance. The most abundant sources of minerals in the plant kingdom are found in sea vegetables: for example nori, hijiki, arame and wakame for their calcium, and dulse for its iron content. Add them in small amounts (about 10–15g/¼–½oz dry weight) to soups, salads and casseroles three to four times a week. Silica, which forms part of the starches that make up hair, is found in common vegetables such as onions, garlic, green leafy vegetables, carrots, cucumber and bell peppers and most sprouted seeds.

Finally, growth rate of hair depends on the kidneys. If your kidneys are strong, your hair will be strong. Healthy kidneys produce lots of fast-growing healthy hair. I can almost guarantee it. Therefore, take care of your kidneys by (1) drinking adequate amounts of water, (2) avoiding salt and the nasty foods (see page 74), and (3) eating foods that strengthen kidney function (see page 40).

HEALTHY NAIL CARE PLAN

A healthy nail should be strong, flexible, pink in color and blemish free. Any change to the surface is a sure sign that something is out of balance. Common signs of nutritional deficiencies include:

- ► Thin and brittle
- ► Splitting
- ► Hard/thick
- ► Peeling
- ► Poor growth
- ► Very pale or transparent
- ► White spots
- ► Vertical ridges
- ► Horizontal ridges
- ► Hang nails
- ► Fungus

NUTRITIONAL SUPPLEMENTS

Nails are affected by a number of conditions, but the most influential is diet. The structure of the nails is made up largely of a protein called keratin and a combination of minerals, including calcium, sulfur, potassium, selenium and other trace elements. Strong, healthy nails are therefore dependent on the sufficient intake of such key minerals.

For tip-top nail care, ensure adequate amounts of protein in your diet. In my practice I use spirulina, blue-green micro algae from the sea, as an efficient source of digestible protein. Its protein digestibility is rated at 85 percent as compared to only 20 percent for meat. It also contains a combination of minerals, beta-carotene and essential fatty acids.

Supplement your diet with royal jelly, high in B vitamins and essential fatty acids. Additional zinc (15–30mg daily) can be incorporated, especially if your nails exhibit white marks or flecks. Silica, a mineral that enhances calcium absorption, is essential. The herb horsetail contains significant amounts of silica and calcium, and can be brewed into a tea three times a day. B complex (50mg a day), borage oil, a rich source of gamma-linolenic acid (GLA), and kelp are all beneficial.

Finally, there is a strong connection between the health of your nails and your liver. If your liver blood is healthy, your nails will be strong. The nails are also a key reflection of the condition of your liver. If the nails are weak or show signs of abnormality, it could mean a problem with this vital organ. To give your liver a boost, implement a diet low in fat, avoid alcohol and drink fresh juices that help purify the liver, including aloe vera, beetroot, cucumber, carrot and apple. (Also see page 108 for foods to nourish the liver.)

Lustrous hair and firm nails are now within easy reach.

TEETH AND GUMS

Hormonal imbalances, mineral deficiencies and poor dental hygiene make gums susceptible to bleeding. Teeth too are put under strain, often caused by mineral depletion. If your teeth or gums have been affected, start strengthening them as soon as possible with appropriate foods and supplements.

Teeth require similar nutrition as you would need for strong bones. Calcium can be obtained from sesame seeds, quinoa, dark leafy greens, seaweed, dried figs and soy foods. Although milk or dairy products contain significant amounts of calcium, they are insufficiently assimilated by the human body and best replaced with plant sources. Magnesium, silica and other vital minerals for teeth are found in most vegetables and whole grains.

HEALTHY TEETH PROGRAM

Here is the program which provides great success to my own patients for healthy teeth and gums.

1 **HERBS**
- Horsetail (2 capsules a day)
- Oatstraw (2 capsules a day)

2 **HERB TEAS**
Choose from comfrey, tea tree, myrrh, licorice, sage, goldenseal and peppermint. Drink 2 or 3 cups a day of the same herb and then rotate to another herb the next day. So you might start with 2 cups of goldenseal tea on Monday, then move on to 2 cups of sage tea on a Tuesday, and so on.

3 **NUTRIENTS**
- Vitamin C with bioflavonoids (1000mg a day)
- Zinc (15–30mg a day)
- Coenzyme Q10 (30mg a day)

4 **TIPS**
- Brush your teeth gently after each meal
- Floss every day
- Rinse with a natural mouthwash that contains one or more of the herbs (herb teas) mentioned in points 1 and 2.

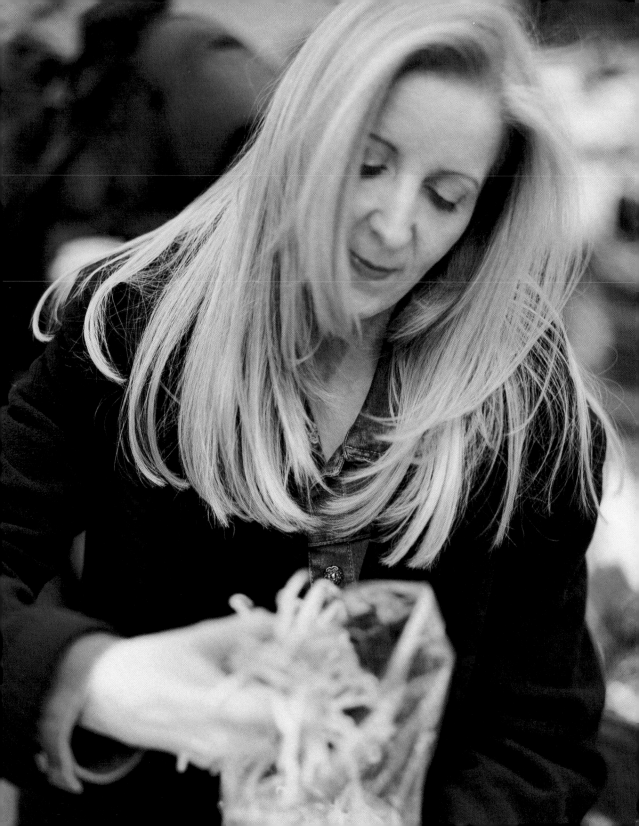

GREAT SEX

Foods can charge up your sexual energy and enhance potency and fertility. The best way to improve your sex life is by looking at your lifestyle – and the cornerstone of your lifestyle is what you eat. If you don't eat good foods, you will experience a decrease in libido, as nutritional deficiencies and poor eating habits adversely affect your hormones, glands and organs. But with just a little care you can easily eat your way back to a great sex life.

I've compiled a list of specific extra-sexy foods. Don't eat them exclusively at the expense of other foods – simply incorporate them into your (hopefully healthy) daily diet and lifestyle. And remember, when you eat for great sex you'll be eating for great health too!

SEXY FOOD LIST

- Aduki beans
- Apples
- Artichokes
- Asparagus
- Avocados
- Bananas
- Beetroot
- Black beans
- Blackberries
- Blackcurrants
- Blueberries
- Brazil nuts
- Brown rice
- Cardamom
- Celery
- Cherries
- Chives
- Chlorella
- Cinnamon
- Daikon root
- Dates
- Dulse seaweed
- Fava beans
- Fennel
- Figs
- Flax/linseeds
- Garlic
- Ginger
- Gooseberries
- Hazelnuts
- Leeks
- Licorice
- Mangos
- Mung beans
- Nori seaweed
- Nutmeg
- Oats
- Okra
- Onions
- Parsley
- Pomegranates
- Pumpkin
- Pumpkin seeds
- Quinoa
- Raspberries
- Saffron
- Seaweed
- Sesame seeds
- Soaked almonds
- Soybeans
- Spinach
- Spirulina
- Sprouted quinoa
- Squash seeds
- Steamed kale
- Strawberries
- Sunflower seeds
- Tomatoes
- Trout
- Turmeric
- Vanilla
- Watercress
- Wild salmon

AND THE SEXIEST FOOD OF ALL IS ...

According to German research, raw sauerkraut. I promise! Watch your lovemaking antics soar once you start eating raw sauerkraut twice a day!

7-DAY JUMPSTART PLAN

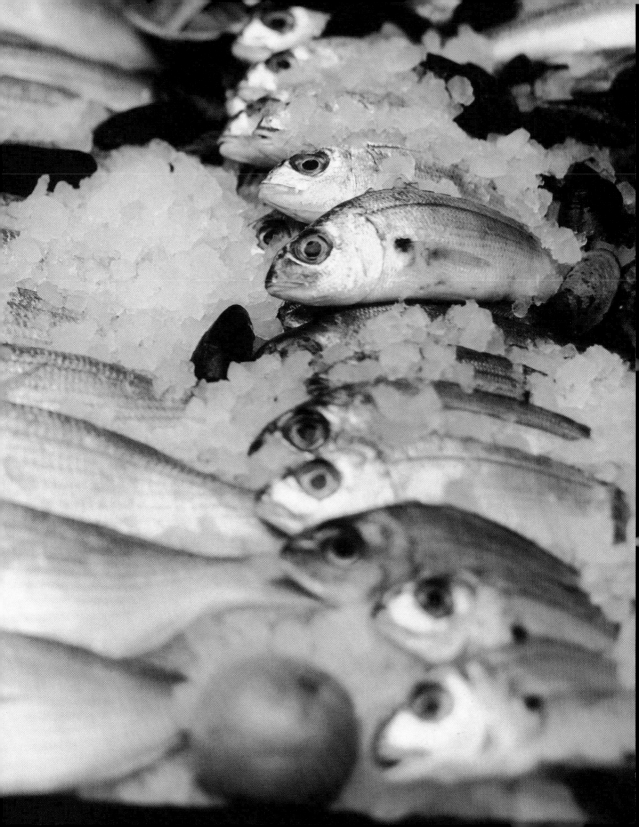

I HAVE DEVISED A SIMPLE PLAN TO HELP
YOU KICKSTART YOUR TRANSFORMATION. BY
READING THE PREVIOUS CHAPTERS YOU'LL NOW
HAVE A REALLY GOOD IDEA ABOUT WHAT'S GOOD
FOR YOU AND WHAT'S NOT, BUT BEFORE YOU GET
INTO THE 7-DAY PLAN, HERE IS SOME GENERAL
ADVICE SO YOU KNOW WHAT TO BUY AND WHAT
TO AVOID IN THE SUPERMARKET.

HOW TO SHOP

A diet high in nutrients and low in additives and preservatives is the key
to good health, but supermarkets can be confusing places with so many
different types of foods, labels and brands. Use the following as a guide
to help choose which foods to include and which to avoid to maintain
good health.

When you walk through the supermarket, aim for the produce aisles
first. This is an aisle bursting with energy from the raw, unadulterated fruit
and vegetables, the way nature intended. Go for what you desire. If you feel
like buying a pint of strawberries, go for it. Which foods speak to you?
Often, if your body needs something, you will start to think of the food that
will take care of that need. Seek out those fruits and vegetables that seem
to be the healthiest, that look in the best condition. Squeeze the peaches
for softness. Examine the apples for blemished skins or holes. Do not buy
or eat old, decrepit looking, wilted fruits or vegetables. They will have no
life force and little nutrient content.

*Note: It's always a good move to choose food that is organically produced
as it has fewer chemicals and additives.*

CANNED BEANS

- ► Choose beans cooked without animal fat or salt.
- ► Avoid canned beans with sugar, salt or preservatives and frozen beans.

WHY? Beans are a fantastic source of nutrients that can help reduce cholesterol but their nutritional value can be depleted if they are canned or cooked in fat and salt. Canned beans are more likely to be high in toxic preservatives and additives. Beans cooked in saturated fats and salt can counteract the cholesterol-lowering effect of beans and increase the risk of heart disease, fluid retention and high blood pressure.

BEVERAGES

- ► Choose herbal teas, fresh (preferably organic) fruits and vegetables and fruit juices, cereal grain beverages, mineral or distilled water.
- ► Avoid alcoholic drinks, coffee, cocoa, pasteurized or sweetened juices, fruit juices, sodas and teas.

WHY? Your body is made up of two-thirds water and water is essential for all bodily functions so it is important to keep your liquid intake high. Pure water is the best drink for quenching thirst and hydrating the body, but don't forget that fruits and vegetables consist of 90 percent water. Alcohol and caffeinated beverages deplete your body of essential nutrients so best to avoid.

DAIRY PRODUCTS

- ► Choose non-fat cottage cheese, unsweetened yogurt, goat's milk and cheese, skim milk, buttermilk, rice milk and all soy products.
- ► Avoid soft, pasteurized or artificially colored cheeses and ice cream.

WHY? Dairy products are a good source of protein but soft cheeses, ice cream and artificially colored cheese products are high in saturated fat, dyes and preservatives. Best to choose the low-fat, additive-free alternatives.

EGGS

- ► Choose organic free-range if possible. When cooking, best to boil or poach.
- ► Avoid fried or pickled.

WHY? Fried or pickled eggs are high in cholesterol-raising saturated fat. Best to avoid. Organic eggs won't contain the toxic hormones and antibiotics pumped into factory-produced eggs.

FISH

- ► Choose all freshwater white fish, salmon, boiled or baked fish, tuna.
- ► Avoid all fried fish, all shellfish, salted fish, anchovies, herring, and fish canned in salt and oil.

WHY? Freshwater and oily fish are rich in the good fats, known as omega-3, essential for reducing cholesterol and promoting health and well-being. They are also low in salt, saturated fat and nutrient-depleting additives.

If possible choose glass bottles. Cans of fizzy drink contain six times the amount of aluminium compared to the same drinks in a glass bottle. There is always a certain amount of residue that dissolves into a drink from the lining of a can or from a plastic bottle so always best to choose glass bottles.

FRUITS

► Choose all fresh, frozen, stewed or dried fruits without sweeteners, unsulfured fruits, home-canned fruits. Try to buy organic where possible.

► Avoid canned, bottled or frozen fruits with sweeteners added.

WHY? Fruits are high in essential fiber, vitamins, minerals and antioxidants. Always best to eat them fresh, because when they are processed or juiced their nutrient and fiber content decreases and their sugar and additive content increases.

GRAINS

► Choose all whole grains and products containing whole grains; cereals, breads, muffins, whole-grain crackers, cream of wheat or rye cereal, buckwheat, millet, oats, brown rice, wild rice.

► Avoid all white flour products, white rice and white pasta.

WHY? Grains are a great energy source, high in energy-releasing nutrients that feed your cells. Whole grains don't have the additives and preservatives that white products do and give you a sustained burst of energy instead of a roller coaster of highs and lows. Unlike white products, whole grains are also rich in fiber which is essential for healthy digestion.

NUTS

► Go for all fresh, raw nuts.

► Avoid salted or roasted nuts.

WHY? Nuts are a good source of protein but you don't need the extra salt, fat and preservatives that go with salted and roasted nuts.

MEATS

► Choose organic skinless turkey, lamb and chicken.

► Avoid beef, all forms of pork, hot dogs, luncheon meats, smoked, pickled and processed meats, corned beef, duck, goose, spare ribs, gravies and organ meats.

WHY? Red meats are high in saturated fat. Factory-farmed meat and poultry often contain hormones and antibiotics that upset your hormonal, immune and digestive systems. Bear in mind too that many processed meats/foods not only are high in additives but also come in packages ready to warm for heating. They are stored wrapped in plastic and aluminium which adds additional non-food chemicals into your food, especially when heated.

OILS

► Choose all cold-pressed oils: corn, safflower, sesame, olive, flaxseed, soybean, sunflower and canola oils; margarine made from these oils, and eggless mayonnaise.

► Avoid all saturated fats, hydrogenated margarine, refined processed oils, shortenings and hardened oils.

WHY? Saturated fats contain substances that encourage blood clotting and inflammation and help raise cholesterol. Processed oils are also high in additives which can harm your health. Cold-pressed oils don't contain these substances or as many additives and are rich in health-boosting essential fatty acids.

SEASONINGS

▸ Choose garlic, onions, cayenne, herbs, dried vegetables, apple cider vinegar, tamari, miso, seaweed and dulse.

▸ Avoid black or white pepper, salt, hot red peppers, all types of vinegar except pure natural apple cider vinegar or rice vinegar.
WHY? Salt causes fluid retention and can raise blood pressure. Instead of salt, experiment with preservative- and additive-free alternatives, such as garlic, thought to reduce cholesterol, and seaweed, packed with minerals and providing incredible health benefits.

SOUPS

▸ Choose salt- and fat-free bean, lentil, pea, vegetable, barley, brown rice and onion homemade fresh soups.

▸ Avoid canned soups made with salt, preservatives, MSG or fat stock and all creamed soups.
WHY? Many canned soups are high in toxic additives and preservatives and contain substances which block the absorption of cholesterol-lowering essential fatty acids. There are some varieties of canned soups which do not contain added chemicals and salt. Also, check in the fridge sections for fresh soups.

SPROUTS AND SEEDS

▸ Choose all types of sprouts, wheatgrass and all raw seeds.

▸ Avoid all seeds cooked in oil or salt.
WHY? Sprouts and seeds are nutritional powerhouses. The majority of these nutrients are destroyed when they are cooked in oil, or when additives and salt are added.

SWEETS

▸ Choose barley malt or rice syrup, raw honey, pure maple syrup, blackstrap molasses that is unsulfured.

▸ Avoid white, brown, or raw cane sugar, corn syrups, chocolate, sugar candy, fructose, all syrups (except pure maple), all sugar substitutes, jams and jellies made with sugar.
WHY? Sugar and sweets high in sugar have no nutritional value and are packed with calories, additives, colorings and preservatives. You don't need them.

VEGETABLES

▸ Choose all raw, fresh, fresh-frozen and preferably organic vegetables.

▸ Avoid all canned or frozen with salt or additives.
WHY? Too much salt added to your vegetable intake can raise your blood pressure. Additives added to canned or frozen vegetables can deplete essential nutrients called phytochemicals – substances that have incredible benefits for your heart, skin, hair and mental and reproductive health. Fresh, raw vegetables contain no additives or preservatives and are therefore higher in health-boosting phytochemicals.

You will find a full selection of the nuts, seeds, beans, grains, pulses, sprouts and legumes I recommend in your local health food store. These stores will also stock lots of vitamin supplements, minerals, herbal teas and superfoods. They often stock alternatives to lots of conventional products too, and pride themselves on offering foods which are organic, chemical- and preservative-free and beneficial to health. And if it all looks pretty confusing, just ask.

READ THE LABELS

It's important to pay attention to food labels and get used to spotting hidden ingredients. Additives in our food have been linked to a variety of health problems including headaches, asthma, allergies, hyperactivity in kids and even cancer. These additives in the form of colorings, preservatives, flavor enhancers, emulsifiers and thickeners can make your body's own detox system less efficient and increase the toxic load.

We are fortunate today that food manufacturers are required to list the ingredients in their products. Despite this, studies show that food labels can still be confusing and misleading for consumers. Look out for the following.

COLORINGS

A dangerous class of additives, and one of the easiest to avoid, are the dyes capable of interacting with and damaging your immune system, speeding up aging and even pushing you in the direction of cancer. Steer clear of foods made with artificial colors. Watch out for labels with any of the following: artificial color added, the words green, blue or yellow followed by a number, color added with no explanation, such as tartrazine (E102), Quinoline yellow (E104), Sunset yellow (E110), Beetroot red (E162), Caramel (E150) or FD and C red no 3.

Some foods contain natural colors obtained from plants and these are safe. The most common is annatto, from the reddish seed of a tropical tree. Annatto is often added to cheese to make it more orange or butter to make it more yellow. Red pigments obtained from beets, green from chlorella and carotene from carrots are also okay.

PRESERVATIVES

The main function of preservatives is to extend a food's shelf life. Citric acid and ascorbic acid (vitamin C, ascorbates, E300-4) are natural antioxidants added to a number of foods and they are safe, but synthetic additives such as BHA and BHT (E320-21) may not be. They may promote the carcinogenic changes in cells caused by other substances.

Alum, an aluminium compound, is used in brands of many pickles to increase crispiness and is also found in some antacids and baking powder. Aluminium has no place in human nutrition and you should avoid ingesting it.

Nitrates (Nitrites, E249-52) are a type of preservative often added to processed meats, such as hot dogs, bacon and ham. They can create highly carcinogenic substances called nitrosamines in the body. It is best to avoid any products containing sodium nitrate or other nitrates.

Monosodium glutamate (MSG or 621) – a natural product used in East Asian cooking – is added to many manufactured foods as a flavor enhancer. It is an unnecessary source of additional sodium in the diet and can cause allergic reactions. Omit MSG from recipes, don't buy products containing it and when eating Chinese request that food be made without it. Other flavor enhancers and preservatives to avoid include monopotassium glutamate (622) and sodium osinate (631) and benzoic acid and benzoates (E210-9) found in soft drinks, beer and salad dressings.

EMULSIFIERS, STABILIZERS AND THICKENERS

These are often found in sauces, soups, breads, cookies, cakes, frozen desserts, ice cream, margarine and other spreads, jams, chocolate and milk shakes.

More and more manufacturers are cleaning up their products as people get more concerned about toxins in their food and you will increasingly see "no artificial sweeteners" or "no artificial ingredients." This is helpful, but watch out still for hidden fats, salts and sugars and alternative names for foods that aren't very good for you when eaten in excess. Sugar, for example, has lots of different names and they include: sucrose, fructose, dextrose, corn syrup, maltodextrin, golden syrup and so on.

Sodium is just another name for salt. Animal fat is saturated fat and trans-fatty acid is another name for hydrogenated fat. Mannitol, sorbitol, xylitol, saccharine and aspartame are alternative names for potentially carcinogenic artificial sweeteners.

Some chemicals are harmless, for instance, ammonium bicarbonate, malic acid, fumaric acid, lactic acid, lecithin, xanathan, guar gums, calcium chloride, monocalcium phosphate and monopotassium phosphate. But how can you tell when there is a long list of long chemical names that look unfamiliar to you? If that's the case, a good general rule is simply to avoid products whose chemical ingredients outnumber the familiar ones.

MEAL PLANNER

THIS MEAL PLANNER WILL HELP YOU GET STARTED. YOU CAN FOLLOW IT TO THE LETTER, OR SIMPLY USE IT AS A FOUNDATION FOR IDEAS. SEE PAGE 82 FOR MY ABUNDANT FOOD LIST TO SLOT IN YOUR OWN IDEAS.

DAY

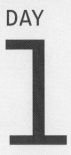
1234567

7:00am
Good morning exercise (page 190)

7:15am
1 cup of warm water with a squeeze of lemon
1 cup nettle tea

7:30am
Go out for a fast brisk 30-minute walk –
work up a sweat.

8:15am BREAKFAST
Large pint of blueberries. Mix with
some raspberries if you so desire.
(If you want a second pint, go for it).

10:15am MID-MORNING SNACK
1 cupful of steamed raw almonds (steam for
2 minutes) and 3 or more stalks of celery

12pm
Go out for a fast 20-minute walk.

12:30pm LUNCH
Tuna fish on a salad bed of spinach
(If you wish, steam the spinach for 1 minute.)
Hold the mayo
6 cherry tomatoes
Heap spinach leaves
Handful of dill herb sprinkled throughout
Squeeze raw lemon and/or a dash of orange

3:00pm MID-AFTERNOON SNACK
Steamed almonds
1 whole raw red pepper

6:00pm
Dance to loud music for 20 minutes before dinner.
Go wild!

6:30pm DINNER
Small veggie juice:
1 cucumber and 1 celery stalk
Miso soup with tofu pieces and scallions
(You can buy miso in packages – just add hot water
and a few chopped spring onions.)
Organic turkey or organic chicken with steamed
carrots and broccoli and a tablespoon of miso soup
to moisten your white meat
Big handful mung bean sprouts and herbal leaves
If you are vegetarian, try my Sweet Potato
Shepherd's Pie (page 186).

8:30–9:00pm
Good night exercise (page 191)

9:00pm EVENING SNACK
1 or 2 fresh raw peaches.

1234567

7:00am
Good morning exercise (as before)

7:15am
1 cup of warm water with a squeeze of lemon
1 cup dandelion tea

7:30pm
Go out for a brisk 30-minute walk.

8:15am BREAKFAST
1 bowl of any type of melon or pineapple
Follow with a bowl of Quinoa Porridge
(page 186).

10:15am MID-MORNING SNACK
Pumpkin seeds and one or more whole
cucumbers with the skin left on

12pm
Go for a fast 20-minute walk.

12:30pm LUNCH
1 or 2 whole soft, ripe avocados sliced up
on a bed of the leftover quinoa from the morning
Decorate with pumpkin seeds and 1 tablespoon
of flax seeds and serve with a heaped handful or
more of raw or lightly steamed green beans.

3:00pm MID-AFTERNOON SNACK
1 or more whole raw yellow peppers

6:00pm
Dance for 20 minutes.

6:30pm DINNER
Aduki Bean Casserole (page186) with squash
and yams, and add a load of alfalfa sprouts when
you serve. Serve with Millet Mash and Onion
Gravy (page 186). Make a big pot as it could serve
for lunch the next day.

8:30pm
Good night exercise (as before)

9:00pm EVENING SNACK
Handful of raw hazelnuts. If you soak hazelnuts for
a couple of hours they will be really easy to digest.

1234567

7:00am
Good morning exercise (as before)

7:15 am
1 cup of warm water with a squeeze of lemon
1 cup fennel tea

7:30am
Brisk 30-minute walk

8:15am BREAKFAST
Blend 1 mango, 1 peach and 1 banana.
Pour over a basket of raspberries.

10:15am MID-MORNING SNACK
A large handful of brazil nuts

12pm:
Get outside for a fast 20-minute walk.

12:30pm LUNCH
Haricot Bean Salad (page 187) or Aduki Bean
Casserole, left over from last night. Serve on
a bed of dark green leafies.

3:00pm MID-AFTERNOON SNACK
Small container of cherry tomatoes
1 chopped fennel

6:00pm
Dance for 20 minutes.

6:30pm DINNER
Lemon sole (or any fresh fish you fancy) with
steamed florets of broccoli, carrots and a basil
bed under the fish. Serve with raw snowpeas.

8:30pm
Good night exercise (as before)

9:00pm EVENING SNACK
1 or more apples

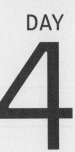

DAY
1 2 3 4 5 6 7

7:00am
Good morning exercise (as before)

7:15am
1 cup of warm water with a squeeze of lemon
1 cup nettle tea

7:30am
Jump up and down on your trampoline
for 15–20 minutes or go for a brisk walk.

8:15am BREAKFAST
Big bunch of grapes
$\frac{1}{2}$ hour later, bowl of porridge oats

10:15am MID-MORNING SNACK
Handful or more of red grapes or cherries

12pm
Go outside for a brisk 15-minute walk.

12:30pm LUNCH
Broccoli Soup (page 187), with a beet salad
made with chicory, avocado, fine celery stalks,
clover sprouts, lettuce, mustard leaves and
radishes. Sprinkle with 2 teaspoons of sesame
seeds, a squeeze of lemon and a few drops of
wheat-free tamari sauce.

3:00pm MID-AFTERNOON SNACK
Bowl of raw sauerkraut, sprinkled with sunflower
or flax seeds

6:00pm
Dance to music for 20 minutes.

6:30pm DINNER
Mung Bean Casserole (page 187) with
Gourmet Brown Rice (page 187). Serve on a
salad leaf bed with a handful of clover sprouts.

8:30pm
Good night exercise (as before)

9:00pm EVENING SNACK
A few whole dates

1234567

7:00am
Good morning exercise (as before)

7:15am
1 cup of warm water with a squeeze
of lemon
1 cup dandelion tea

7:30 am
Brisk 30-minute walk

8:00am BREAKFAST
Fruit Salad of fresh peaches, pears and
strawberries, sprinkled with mint leaves
1/2 hour later, bowl of barley in miso broth

10:15am MID-MORNING SNACK
2 or more carrots

12pm
Brisk 20-minute walk before lunch

12:30 LUNCH
Squash and Sweet Potato Soup (page 187).
If you need to eat more after that, then go
for a chickpea, chicory and fennel salad,
served with a generous portion of lightly
steamed beans and sprouted alfalfa seeds.
Thin slices of carrot to garnish.

3:00pm MID-AFTERNOON SNACK
1 or more whole cucumbers

6:00pm
Jump and down on your trampoline to music
for 20 minutes.

6:30pm DINNER
Veggie Sushi Rolls (page 188) with
a heaped handful of sprouted clover
and sprouted sunflower seeds. Serve
with sauerkraut.

8:30pm
Good night exercise (as before)

9:00pm EVENING SNACK
Celery sticks: Dip into avocado sauce.

7:00am
Good morning exercise (as before)

7:15am
1 cup of warm water with a squeeze of lemon
1 cup fennel tea

7:30am
Brisk 30-minute walk

8:00am
Celery, cucumber and carrot juice
$1/2$ hour later, bowl of Quinoa Porridge (page 186)

10:15am MID-MORNING SNACK
Pint of blueberries

12pm
Brisk 20-minute walk before lunch

12:30pm LUNCH
Hearty Lentil Stew (page 188) with a generous
handful of bean sprouts

3:00pm MID-AFTERNOON SNACK
2 raw carrots
1 whole raw yellow pepper

6:00pm
Skipping rope for 10 minutes
Jump up and down on your trampoline
for 10 minutes.

6:30pm DINNER
Marinated Baked Wild Salmon with Vitality Salad
(page 188)

8:30pm
Good night exercise (as before)

9:00pm EVENING SNACK
Bean sprouts and celery sticks with vegetable dip
(page 189)

7:15am
Good morning exercise (as before)

7:30am
1 cup of warm water with a squeeze of lemon

8:00am
Brisk 30-minute walk

8:30am BREAKFAST
Dr. Gillian's Berry Blast:
1 pint strawberries and 1 banana
Blend until smooth
Add 1 tablespoon of whole blueberries and
3 heaped teaspoons of Dr. Gillian's Living
Food Energy Powder (see page 220).

10:15am MID-MORNING SNACK
Veggie juice:
1 cucumber, 4 celery stalks, 1/2 apple,
a few sprigs of mint, dill or basil, plus
1 teaspoon of spirulina mixed in

12pm
Vigorous 20-minute walk

12:30pm LUNCH
Turnip and Leek Soup (page 189),
sprinkled with lots of sprouted seeds
and raw parsley. Alternatively try my
Baked Veggie Bean Burger (page 189).

1:30pm
Veggie juice:
Cucumber Medley (page 145)

3:00pm MID-AFTERNOON SNACK
Veggie juice:
1 cucumber, 4 celery stalks, 1/2 beet and
a small piece of ginger

6:00pm
Gentle exercise. Walk for 30 minutes.

6:30pm DINNER
Lots of chicory leaves filled with
tabbouleh (page 188). Garnish with
a few chopped up brazil nuts.

9:00pm EVENING SNACK
2 or more pears

RECIPES

CHICKEN DELIGHT
(SERVES 2)

2 chicken breasts (or turkey)
Handful of basil leaves
8 cherry tomatoes
Miso or bouillon (1/2 cup)
Handful of mung bean sprouts
or fresh herbs
2 handfuls of green salad leaves
Handful of spinach

Lay a sheet of foil in a baking tray
and place the chicken breasts on the
foil. Tear the basil leaves, halve the
tomatoes and toss over the chicken.
Using a teaspoon of bouillon or miso,
mix with a half cup of boiling water to
make a stock and then pour over the
chicken. Fold over the foil to make a
parcel and bake in the oven on 400°F
for 20 minutes.

Serve the chicken on a bed of raw
or lightly steamed spinach with a salad
made from the fresh herbs, mung
sprouts and salad leaves.

QUINOA PORRIDGE
(SERVES 1)

2 cups water
1 cup quinoa grain
Pinch of bouillon powder

Boil the water and then add the quinoa.
Season with a pinch of bouillon powder
(don't use table salt). Bring water back
to boil and simmer on low heat for
approximately 7 minutes. Switch off
and let sit for 15 minutes.

SWEET POTATO SHEPHERD'S PIE
(SERVES 4)

2 tsp virgin olive oil
1 garlic clove, peeled and crushed
1 onion, peeled and sliced
2 sticks celery, washed and sliced
1 bay leaf
1 small butternut squash, peeled,
halved, deseeded and cut into small
pieces
15oz vegetable stock (made with 1
vegetable stock cube or your own
stock)
15oz can "no added salt" red kidney
beans, rinsed in a colander under cold
running water and drained
2 red or yellow peppers, washed,
deseeded and sliced
4 tomatoes, washed and sliced in half
2 medium zucchini, sliced
1 broccoli head, finely chopped
3 medium carrots, sliced
2 tbsp finely chopped fresh parsley
1 tsp arrowroot
4 sweet potatoes, steamed for 15
minutes until soft, and mashed

Heat a little water and the olive oil
in a large saucepan. Add the garlic,
onion, celery and bay leaf and simmer
for approximately 3 minutes. Add the
squash and heat for further 3 minutes,
stirring. Pour in the stock and bring
to a boil over a medium heat. Simmer
gently for 10 minutes, stirring
occasionally. Add the kidney beans,
peppers, tomatoes, zucchini, broccoli,
and carrots. Simmer for a further 5
minutes until the squash is just tender.
Stir in the parsley. Add a little
arrowroot to thicken.

Transfer into a baking dish, mix the
sweet potato mash with a little of the
cooking water and a dash of tamari
sauce and add as a topping and bake
for 15 minutes at 400°F. Just enough
to set.

ADUKI BEAN CASSEROLE
(SERVES 4)

1 cup aduki beans (soak for 2 hours
before cooking)
1 vegetable stock cube
1 tbsp miso paste
1 small squash, roughly chopped
2 carrots
1 onion, peeled and sliced
1 handful chervil
1 handful sprouted seeds
1 head chicory
1 radish per chicory leaf

Use 1 cup aduki beans to 3 cups water.
Add the veggie stock cube to the
water, bring to a boil and simmer for
30 minutes. (If you add a strip of the
seaweed kombu to the stew, it adds lots
of fantastic nutrients to your meal.
Rinse one strip under water and add to
stew. You don't have to eat the seaweed
to get the nutrients.) Halfway through
the 30 minutes, add the squash. At the
end of the 30 minutes, add the onion
and carrots and stir in miso. Add the
chervil and garnish with chicory,
sprouted seeds and radishes.

MILLET MASH
(SERVES 4)

1 cup millet
1 small cauliflower, thinly sliced
2 1/2 cups water
Pinch of sea salt
1/4 cup fresh parsley, chopped

Wash the millet and drain well. Add
a pinch of salt to the water and bring
to a boil. Thinly slice the cauliflower,
then add to the water along with the
millet. Bring to a boil and then
reduce heat and simmer for 20
minutes. Remove from the heat and
mash well with a potato masher. Fold
parsley in just before serving.

ONION GRAVY
(SERVES 4)

2 large onions, peeled and thinly sliced
1 tsp olive oil
2 cups springwater
2 tsp wheat-free tamari sauce
Thickener (1 tsp arrowroot)

Peel and slice the onions. Warm the oil in a pan with a little water and add the onions. Simmer for 15 minutes on a low temperature. Add the springwater. Combine the tamari and arrowroot with enough cold water to dissolve. Add this mixture to onion-and-water mix and stir over a medium heat until thick and clear. Blend for a smooth gravy.

Alternatively you can use a miso soup pack. Simply add boiling water to the powder and use as gravy over the millet mash.

CREAMY BROCCOLI SOUP
(SERVES 4)

3 heads of broccoli, chopped
6 cups of water or more (enough to cover the vegetables)
1 whole fennel, diced
1 vegetable bouillon cube
Handful of fresh tarragon and handful of fresh sage leaves
1 cup of fresh sprouts

Boil water, add the broccoli and simmer for 7 minutes. Turn off the heat and add all other ingredients except the sprouts. Blend in a food processor. You may adjust soup consistency by adding more or less water. Add the sprouts into the blender once everything else is blended, or serve soup with whole sprouts as garnish. You can vary the recipe by using different types of herbs such as fresh parsley, coriander or dill.

MUNG BEAN CASSEROLE
(SERVES 4)

1 cup mung beans
1 vegetable stock cube
1/4 tsp turmeric powder
1/2 tsp coriander powder
1/4 tsp cumin powder
2 carrots
1 onion
1 handful chervil
1 fennel
2 cups kale, steamed for 2–3 mins
1 pinch sea salt

Use 1 cup mung beans to 3 cups water. Add the vegetable stock cube to the water, bring to boil, add sea salt and simmer for 30 minutes. Add the turmeric, coriander and cumin. After the 30 minutes, add the onion and carrots. Decorate with generous amounts of chervil and serve on a bed of fennel, kale and sprouted seeds. Clover sprouts are great.

HARICOT BEAN SALAD
(SERVES 4)

1 can "no added salt" beans
1 celery stick, washed and chopped
3 baby pickles, finely chopped
1 red pepper, sliced
1 yellow pepper, sliced
Sauerkraut and salad leaves
Sprinkle of sunflower seeds
Vinaigrette dressing

Toss all the ingredients together to make this delicious salad.

GOURMET BROWN RICE RECIPE
(SERVES 4)

1 cup brown rice
1 vegetable stock cube
2 carrots
1 onion
1/2 cup fresh peas

Add 1 cup of brown rice to 2 cups of boiling water. Add the stock cube. Simmer for 20 minutes until the rice is tender and almost all of the water has been absorbed but not totally absorbed. Take off the heat and let sit for 10 minutes, when it will be ready to serve. Toss in the peas at the last moment.

SQUASH AND SWEET POTATO SOUP
(SERVES 4)

6–8 cups water
1 vegetable bouillon cube
3 cups butternut squash, cubed
1 fennel
1 cup sweet potatoes or yams, cubed
1 cup carrots, cubed
6–8 onions, sliced
1 handful tarragon and parsley
1 clove garlic
Sprinkle of pumpkin and sesame seeds

Add the stock cube to the water and bring to a boil. Add the squash, fennel, sweet potatoes, carrots and onions and boil lightly for 5–8 minutes, until tender but firm. Take away from heat and add the tarragon, parsley and garlic. Blend in the food processor. Soup may be thicker or thinner depending on the amount of water used. Garnish with chopped up radishes, pumpkin seeds and sesame seeds.

VEGGIE SUSHI ROLLS
(SERVES 4)

2 cups soft mashed avocado or
avocado cream sauce
Raw nori sheets
2 cups brown rice, cooked
Long thin strips cucumber
1 cup shredded carrots
1 cup alfalfa sprouts or sunflower
sprouts or clover sprouts or a
combination
1 cup shredded cabbage
1 onion, diced thinly
Sprinkle of fresh dill

Spread avocado mash onto the nori
sheets (shiny side down). Leave 1 inch
of nori sheet exposed at one end to help
seal the roll. Across the center, place a
row of each of the following: rice,
cucumber, carrot, sprouts, onion,
cabbage, dill. Roll the nori from the
bottom, squeezing tightly. When rolled,
it should be firm and strong.

AVOCADO CREAM SAUCE

2 very soft avocados
2 spring onions, finely chopped
1/4 tsp of coriander powder
1/4 tsp seaweed seasoning (or sea salt)
1/2 tsp olive oil
3–4 tbsp water (preferably still
mineral water)

Place the water at the bottom of a
blender. Add the avocados, spring
onion, coriander, seasoning, olive oil
and mix until smooth and creamy.

HEARTY LENTIL STEW
(SERVES 4)

1 cup lentils, soaked for 20 minutes
and rinsed thoroughly
2 bay leaves
2 onions
1 vegetable bouillon cube
2 cups diced squash
1 sweet potato
4 carrots
1 stalk celery
1 handful watercress
1 tsp wheat-free tamari sauce

Place the lentils, onions and bay leaves
in a pot with 3 cups of water and
stock cube, cover and bring to the boil.
Simmer for 30–35 minutes. Halfway
through, add the squash and sweet
potatoes. After a further 10 minutes,
add the carrots and celery. Toward the
end, add the watercress and stir in the
tamari sauce.

To turn this into soup for the next
day, add more water, extra fresh herbs
of your choice, some more stock and
blend until smooth.

RAW VITALITY SALAD
(SERVES 4)

Generous amount arugala leaves
1 daikon, peeled and sliced
8 cherry tomatoes
1 stalk of celery, chopped
1 yellow zucchini, sliced
6 small radishes chopped into halves
2 tbsp raw sunflower seeds or sesame
seeds or pumpkin seeds
1 handful of mung bean sprouts
2 carrots, grated
1 handful of dill
Squeeze of lemon

Toss all the ingredients together
for this energy-packed salad. Serve
with my Sesame Miso Dressing (see
opposite page).

MARINATED BAKED SALMON
(SERVES 2)

2 leeks
2 salmon steaks
Generous handful spinach
2 cloves garlic, peeled and crushed
2 tbsp olive oil
1 tbsp grated ginger
Juice of 1 lemon
1 cup fresh coriander

Cut the leeks into approximately
12 chunks and steam or boil for about
5 minutes to gently soften. Rinse and
dry the salmon. Place a liberal amount
of fresh raw spinach in a shallow oven
pan. Place the softened leeks on top
of the spinach. Then place the salmon
on top of the leeks. Mix the olive oil,
crushed garlic and grated ginger
together; then brush it over the fish.
Keep some extra olive oil mixture on
hand. Squeeze fresh lemon juice onto
the fish and spinach. Place into
preheated oven at 400°F for
approximately 25 minutes. While
cooking, brush the olive oil mixture
onto the salmon every 10 minutes.
Decorate the plate with coriander
leaves and add a last squeeze of lemon.

TABBOULEH
(SERVES 4)

2/3 cup cooked quinoa
1/2 cup fresh mint, chopped
1 1/2 cups fresh parsley, chopped
1 large tomato, diced
1 medium cucumber, peeled and diced
2/3 cup chopped onions
1 tbsp extra virgin olive oil
1 whole fresh lemon, juiced
1 pinch sea salt

Mix all ingredients together in large
bowl. Cover and chill for 20 minutes.
Serve the tabbouleh mounded on a
bed of lettuce, accompanied by
lemon wedges.

VEGGIE BEAN BURGERS
(MAKES 4 BURGERS)

2 cups cooked beans (use black beans,
aduki, pinto, kidney or chickpeas)
1 cup steamed squash
1 carrot
1/2 onion, finely sliced
1 small shallot
1/2 cup miso liquid or stock liquid
to moisten patties a little
1 tbsp fresh herbs or powdered
(coriander, sage, parsley, thyme,
dill, basil, ginger, fennel, cumin,
mint, garlic are all good choices)
1/2 cup cooked brown rice
Sunflower seeds if you desire

Mash up the beans. Mix in the
other ingredients and make patties.
Bake for 30 minutes at
200°C/400°F/Gas 6 until brown. Serve
with my avocado cream sauce.

TURNIP AND LEEK SOUP
(SERVES 4)

1 bouillon cube
2 small turnips, peeled and diced
6 leeks, sliced
6 stalks celery, chopped
3 onions, finely sliced
1 garlic clove, crushed
1 handful tarragon

Add the stock cube to approximately 1
quart water and bring to a boil. Add the
turnip and simmer for 10 minutes. Add
in the leeks and then boil for further 5
minutes. Add the onions, celery and
garlic and simmer for further 5
minutes. Take off the heat, add the
tarragon and then blend.

TREATS
LEMON PUDDING
(SERVES 1–2)

2 avocados, mashed
1 1/2 cups lemon flesh
1/2 lemon for juice
1/2 pear for juice
2 cups pitted dates
3 tbsp maple syrup
2 tbsp pear juice

Place all ingredients together
and squeeze in the fresh orange
and lemon juices. Then mix in a
blender or food processor.

CAROB FUDGE DELIGHT
(SERVES 4–6)

1 1/4 cup pitted dates
3/4 cup soaked raisins
4 tbsp carob powder
2 cups soaked Brazil nuts
1 cup water
1/2 cup ground flax seeds
1/2 cup ground sunflower seeds
1 cup walnut pieces
Sprinkle of sesame seeds

Blend the dates, raisins, carob, Brazil
nuts and water in a food processor.
Then mix in the seeds along with the
walnut pieces. Spread onto a tray,
freeze and cut into squares. Sprinkle
with sesame seeds.

SESAME MISO DRESSING

1/3 cup sesame or olive oil
3/4 cup water
3 tbsp apple cider vinegar
3 tbsp light yellow miso
1 clove garlic, crushed
1/2 tsp basil
1/2 tsp oregano

Combine all ingredients and mix or
blend until smooth.

DIPS AND SPREADS
GUACAMOLE

1 or 2 ripe avocados, mashed
1/2 lemon, squeezed
1/2 lime, squeezed
1 red pepper, finely chopped
1 tbsp apple cider vinegar
6 small cherry tomatoes
Dill or arugala to garnish

Mash the avocados in a bowl. Add all
of the other ingredients and mix well.

HUMMUS AND TAHINI CAN
ALSO BE USED FOR DIPPING
VEGGIE STICKS.

VEGGIE SPREADS

1 cup cooked veggies or cooked beans
1 handful parsley and chive, chopped
1 pinch coriander
1 tbsp tahini
2 tsp miso paste
1/2 onion, finely chopped

Mash and serve as a spread or dip.

2 cups parsnips, diced (yams or
sweet potatoes fine too)
2 cups carrots
1/2 cup springwater
2 tbsp sesame tahini
1/2 tsp soya or tamari sauce

Steam the vegetables. Purée in a
blender and then add the tahini and
tamari sauce.

GOOD MORNING EXERCISE

The following exercise will help you to become more balanced and energized first thing in the morning. This means you will be calmer, more relaxed, less stressed. As a result your digestion will then work better too, thus making it easier to maintain a healthy body.

STEP ONE: Find Your Emotional Core

It is so easy to lose your original self. All of our emotional holding occurs in our center core. Both the stomach and the colon are in that general core vicinity, just near or at our center. When we have an emotional upset, we tend to block the natural flow of energy that should emanate from our core center. When we sleep, we tend to hold these emotions. We then wake up and often feel tense, agitated, or like we "got out of the wrong side of the bed." We can change all this for the better, and your whole day can be stress-free and loaded with more energy!

So here is all you need to do:

▶ Sit down on a chair (preferably a hard surface chair) with feet firmly flat against the floor. I want you to actually feel the sensation of your feet against the floor. This will help ground you.

▶ Next take your right hand, with full palm open, and place it in on the area just below your navel. That's your center core. Feel your center with your hand for a couple minutes, and listen to your breathing.

▶ You are then free to remove your hand, but continue to think about your center. Just use all of your senses to stay with your core. Sit quietly for one or two minutes and think about your emotional center.

STEP TWO: Free the Energy

This next step just requires that you stay in the chair with feet firmly and flatly planted on the floor as above for another couple more minutes.

▶ Find your emotional center again, using your mind. Then visualize an imaginary thin white light or rodlike beam emanating from your emotional center.

▶ Now visualize the white light moving to the right of the emotional center toward your right leg. The imaginary light will then slowly move down your leg, past the knee, as it keeps traveling toward your right foot.

▶ Once it gets down through your right foot, visualize this beam of light starting to travel toward the left in the open space between your two feet. Thus, the light is now making its way toward the sole of the left foot.

▶ The light starts to travel up the left foot and through the leg, as it slowly passes the left knee, and back up the full left leg. At that point, the light beam begins to move toward the right, into the emotional center again.

▶ You may do this over and over a few times. Please do this exercise in a very slow continuous nonstop flowing movement. My Good Morning Exercise here will help you to be more positive, happier and healthier, with a more balanced natural flow of energy through your system.

GOOD NIGHT EXERCISE

Many new medical and scientific studies now prove that our body's cells and molecules listen to the messages that we express and they respond accordingly. If we constantly tell ourselves negative statements like we are too tired, too old, too ill, can't lose the weight, can't get the job, can't make the money, can't find love, and so on, not only our subconscious but our body's molecules, cells, organs and blood will listen carefully and ultimately adopt the same attitude of downward spiral.

We can create positive cellular and organ response with affirmative, happy, calm and loving messages to our own biochemistry and physiology. Talking nicely to yourself works. When the body is in harmony with itself and its environment, our own energetic flow and healing vibration work like a charm to render a healthy system. Too often we obstruct our own energetic flow and healing capability with negative messages that disrupt the delicate smooth flow of our organs and cells.

So try my Good Night Exercise which will assist digestion, calm the nerves, help burn fats, break down carbs, induce sleep, balance the thyroid, thymus, stomach, bowels, while harmonizing the whole body system, physically, mentally and emotionally. I realize that for many of you, at first it might seem a bit silly. You might even feel a bit uncomfortable. But be open to what I am suggesting. Try it, laugh a little, if you feel so inclined, but do give it a go. This exercise will take less than five minutes.

► Sit down on a hard surface chair in a quiet room by yourself. Have both feet firmly on the ground with your shoes off.

► Close your eyes. Imagine a beautiful white light rod entering your body from above through the top of the head. Slowly, deeply and gently inhale and exhale. Breathe in through the nose and out through the mouth.

► Breathe in deeply. On your first long exhalation quietly and slowly say the words, "I love me." The words almost end up in a hummm as you slowly breathe them out.

► Slowly and deeply inhale again, and on the exhale say the words, "I am a being of love."

► On the next exhale, say, "calm."

► Breathe in again and on the exhale say the words, "I feel fabulous." Say this three times, each time on the exhale.

► You need not try to make anything happen here. You just need to say these words and allow the body to take over. All the while, feel and imagine a beautiful white light shining throughout the insides of your body and emanating outward.

► After the breathing and saying these words, now just remain seated and do nothing. Just be for a couple minutes.

► This entire exercise above can be done in less than 5 minutes total. This is the beauty of it. Never say that you don't have the time. And if you are really enjoying it, I suggest you do this same exercise before each meal, or at least before your biggest meal of the day. Do what feels best for you.

CHAPTER 8

MY 20 SUPER QUICK TIPS

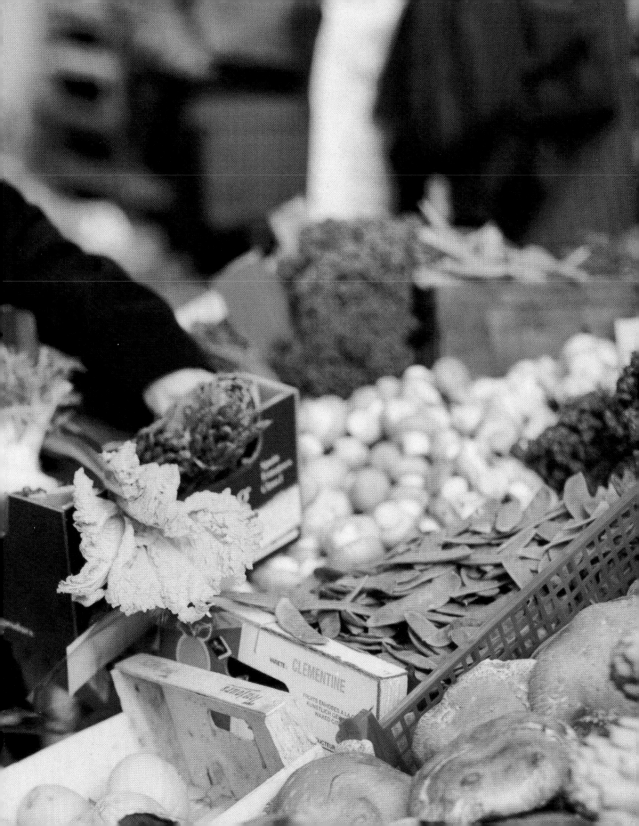

IF THERE'S ONE THING I WANT YOU TO TAKE AWAY FROM THIS BOOK IT'S THAT I'D LIKE YOU TO KEEP THIS CHAPTER READILY AVAILABLE AS A QUICK REFERENCE. THESE 20 SUPER QUICK TIPS, EVEN THOUGH SOME ARE QUITE EASY, COULD TOTALLY CHANGE YOUR LIFE FOREVER. MY PATIENTS ALL TELL ME HOW MUCH THEY HAVE BENEFITED FROM THEM. I AM SURE YOU WILL TOO.

1 DRINK WARM WATER IN THE MORNING

A warm cup of water first thing in the morning (and even better with a squeeze of lemon) goes right through the bowels and cleans mucus out from the day before. Drink another cup of warm water in the evening too.

2 LUBRICATE, DON'T FLOOD

Your stomach needs to be lubricated, not flooded. When you drink fluids with meals, you drown your digestive enzymes and only partial digestion takes place. Therefore, drink fluids, juices, or preferably water, 30 minutes away from meals – say 30 minutes before or after, but not during.

3 CHEW SLOWLY

Chewing slowly until food becomes liquefied is one of my most important recommendations. Really savor each mouthful. Feel the texture and capture the flavor of your food. It's when your saliva comes into contact with your food, as it is being chewed, that the digestive process begins. The chewed food will then pass easily through your digestive system with maximum nutrient uptake.

4 EAT WHEN CALM

You physically can't digest food properly if you are upset or have just had an argument. Eat when calm. Your digestion will be much better.

194

5 NOT TOO HOT – NOT TOO COLD

The temperature of food and drink entering your body affects the strength of your spleen, your energy battery, and other organs too. Ice-cold drinks weaken the organs. Eating piping hot foods that burn your palate aren't much better, since they injure mouth membranes, damage gastric stomach lining and degrade taste buds. Tepid or room temperature foods, drinks and water are best.

6 DECORATE YOUR PLATE

When you smell food, feast your eyes on it or even think about it, your brain is spurred into action, sending a message to the salivary glands to secrete saliva which contains a digestive enzyme. So prepare attractive, delicious meals to enhance your digestion.

7 ROTATE FOODS

Don't eat the same foods every day. You don't need too much of one single food and it can often lead to food allergies, sensitivities and intolerances. So instead eat a particular food just once every four days as opposed to every day. You'll not only prevent allergies, but will also nourish your body with a broader array of varied nutrients.

8 LISTEN TO YOUR BODY

Take note of what foods you crave. If you really want a specific food – its color, the smell or the feel – just enjoy and go with the attractions. It may be that your body needs something nutritionally contained within that food. I'm not talking chocolate cookies here! I'm referring to all those fresh herbs, fruits, vegetables, seasonings and so on that are readily available in any food store or supermarket. Walk the produce aisle for fresh fruits and vegetables with an open mind and an open spirit. What looks good? What feels good? What smells good? Which foods look healthy and robust? Then make your choices.

9 ENZYMES! ENZYMES! ENZYMES!

Sprouted seeds, raw vegetables, raw fruits, nuts and seeds are loaded with live enzymes, the key to nutrient absorption and vibrant health. See page 213 for more information on enzymes and how to sprout your own seeds at home.

10 BREAK THE FAST

Always eat something healthy and substantial for breakfast. This is the time period when your stomach energies are at their strongest, and your digestive enzyme juices are raring to go. You will gradually weaken your stomach and digestive function if you skip breakfast. No matter how little it is, eat something decent. Fresh fruit, oatmeal, millet or quinoa porridge are all good morning choices.

11 NIMBLE AT NIGHT

Eat your last meal of the day at least a couple of hours before bedtime. When you eat too late, you stress and wear out your body. You cannot digest a late meal effectively if you go to sleep on a full stomach. It's bad for your digestive organs, heart and liver, not to mention your libido!

12 CHOOSE CRUCIFEROUS VEGGIES

Eat lots of cabbage, broccoli, Brussels sprouts or cauliflower. These will help you detox and energize your blood.

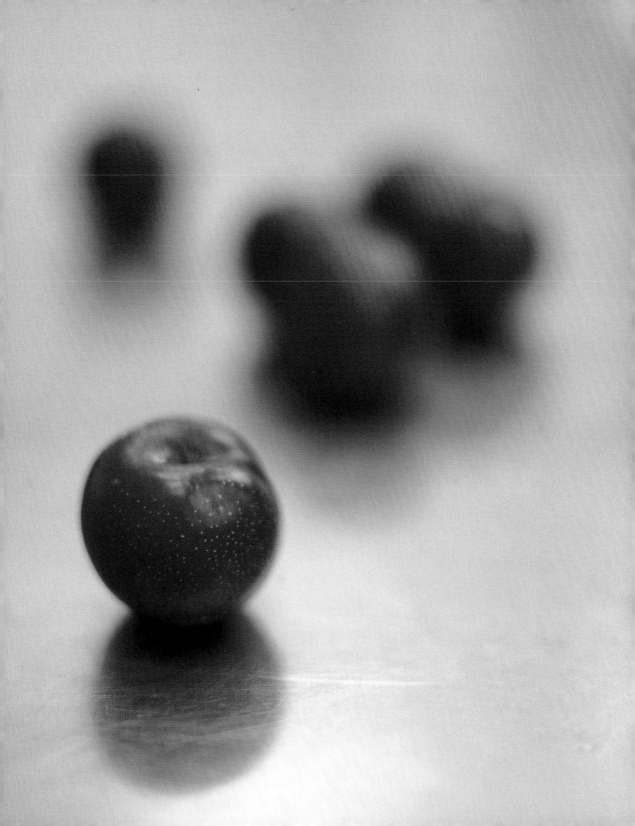

13 DRINK YOUR GREENS

Once a week, make yourself a green juice. Green juices, made from a variety of green vegetables, have a rejuvenating effect on the body because they are rich in chlorophyll (the lifeblood of the plant) which helps to purify the blood, build red blood cells, detoxify the body and provide fast energy. Green juice is the perfect fuel for your body. Its high water content means it is easily assimilated, and it contains the whole vegetable except for the fiber, which is the indigestible part of the plant. Green juice therefore provides all the healthful ingredients in a form that is easy to absorb and digest. Here is just one option, feel free to experiment with your own ideas: 1 carrot, 1 cucumber, 4 celery stalks, 1 fennel stalk, some spinach leaves, a tiny piece of root ginger, a parsley sprig and a handful of alfalfa sprouts (optional). You could also add 1 teaspoon of my Living Food Energy Powder or a superfood green powder to this drink for super results. See page 202 for Superfood Choices.

14 FOOD COMBINE

Fruit + Meat/Fish = Gas
Fruit by Itself = No Gas
In other words, eat foods together that don't compete.
For further details on food combining, see page 78.

15 KIDNEY MASSAGE

The kidneys are the most important organs for overall vitality. At the end of each day, treat yourself to a kidney rub. Before retiring to bed, find your kidneys by placing your hands on your back below the waist, but above your butt. Visualize a warm white light coursing through your body to your hands. Your hands will begin to feel warm as you transfer that heat and light into the kidneys. Massage the kidney region. Then lie down on top of a ready-prepared hot water bottle.

16 MY LITTLE SECRET

I keep a mini trampoline tucked away in the cupboard in the office at my clinic. In between seeing patients and presenting the very dignified health practitioner front, I bring out my mini trampoline and start jumping. The patients never know, because I do it the minute they leave my room. Any form of regular moderate exercise, stretching, walking, bicycling, swimming, tai chi – even dancing – will help move lymph, expel toxins, motivate the blood and revitalize the body.

17 RUB A DUB

At shower/bath time, but *before* you actually get in the bath or shower, take a body cloth, soak it in hot water and rub it all over your body. Start at the feet and work your way up the legs, torso and arms, always toward the heart. This will get your blood moving and spur the energy meridians, improving your digestion.

18 SKIN BRUSH

Brush your skin with a dry skin body brush once weekly to get your lymph moving. See page 163 for more on skin brushing.

19 EARLY TO BED

The earlier you get to bed, the better you will feel. The liver and gallbladder conduct their detox work generally between the hours of 11 P.M. and 2 A.M. If you are not in bed by 11 P.M., you disturb the natural cleansing process, and as a result you will feel sluggish.

20 JUST BE

Take 5 minutes of quiet time each morning to "just be," stop and reflect, before you start rushing for the day. Don't think, don't do, just be. Your eyes can be open or closed, it doesn't matter. But take a few precious moments just for you. Those few valuable minutes will help to balance your biochemistry for the rest of the day.

CHAPTER 9

THE NEXT LEVEL

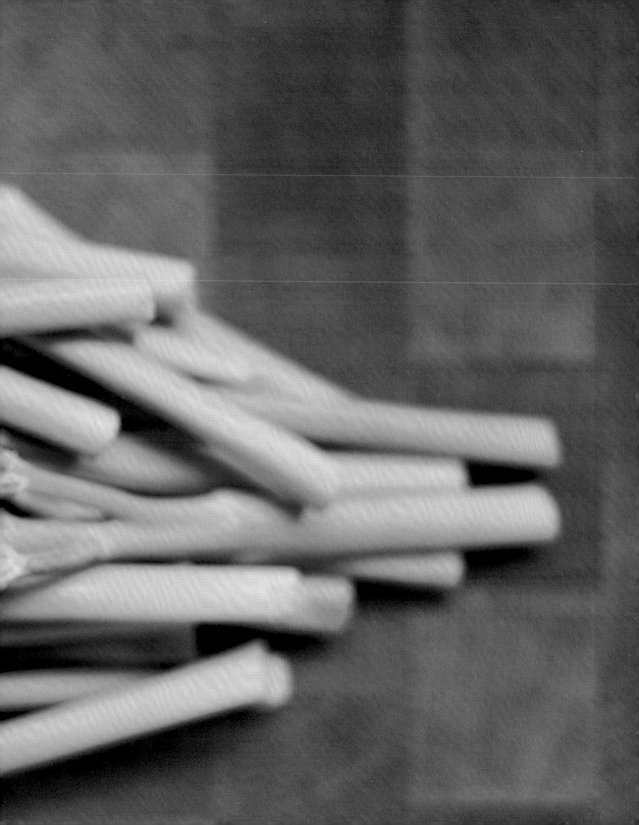

SUPERFOODS
FOR A SUPER BODY

Years ago, when I lived in America, I was very ill and was passed from doctor to doctor. For almost two years, I had suffered with a severe nonstop migraine and a host of other ailments. I used to drag myself out of bed to host a national health radio program. Then one day, a guest on the radio show claimed he had cured himself of cancer using the superfood wild blue-green algae. I initially thought the man was crazy. I would never condone someone refusing hospital treatment but it did inspire me to find this superfood that I had never heard of before. Within three days of taking enormous quantities of wild blue-green algae, just like the radio guest told me to do, my migraine completely disappeared for the first time in two years!

Now as a clinical nutritionist working with patients, I use wild blue-green algae and many other superfoods for excellent results with preventing illness, strengthening the organs, feeding the cells and staying fit, slim and ultra-well. My own little daughters are fed wild blue-green algae throughout the winter to ward off colds and flu. The superfoods are the most powerful nutrient-dense foods on this planet, and they virtually have no calories, no bad fats or nasty substances. Thus, they are powerhouses for any transformation to a slender and more healthy you.

I divide superfoods into five distinct groups:
1 Green superfoods
2 Bee superfoods
3 Herb superfoods
4 Sea vegetables
5 Leafy superfoods

GREEN SUPERFOODS

- ► Alfalfa grass
- ► Green barley grass
- ► Wheatgrass
- ► Wild blue-green algae
- ► Spirulina
- ► Chlorella

WHAT'S SO SPECIAL ABOUT GREEN SUPERFOODS?

They have the best concentration of easily digestible nutrients, fat-burning compounds, vitamins and minerals to protect and heal your body. They also contain a range of other substances including essential fatty acids and healthy bacteria which help your digestive system function more effectively, and protect you against disease and illness.

THE GRASSES

Please note that rotation of the grass juices is recommended for maximum health benefits.

ALFALFA GRASS:
THE FATHER OF ALL FOODS

Alfalfa rejuvenates the whole system by boosting your strength, vigor and vitality. It contains all the known vitamins (four times more vitamin C than citrus fruit) and minerals (a calcium content so high it's off the charts), plus digestive enzymes, phytoestrogen (plant-based hormones), flavonoids, amino acids and chlorophyll.

Alfalfa grass is most commonly used for detoxifying and enriching the liver, assisting weight loss, strengthening and purifying the blood, aiding digestion and as a general tonic, a real boost to the immune system. You can buy alfalfa grass powder in a health food store. It also comes in tablets and capsules too for ease of use.

GREEN BARLEY GRASS:
DETOXER EXTRAORDINAIRE

Barley grass contains just about every nutrient required by the human body, except vitamin D. It's very similar to wheatgrass, and is easy to digest. It's a deep green leafy plant containing nutrients similar to that of leafy green vegetables, but with many times the level of vitamins, minerals and proteins. It has as much protein as meat, and is packed with goodness. Barley grass has eleven times the calcium of cow's milk, five times the iron of spinach, and seven times more vitamin C than orange juice. Barley grass is beneficial for all tissues and organs, especially the heart, lungs, arteries, joints and bones.

When it comes to the health advantages of barley grass, how long have you got? They're almost too numerous to list but here are a few anyway. It helps protect against pollutants, radiation, cancer, ulcers and digestive problems. It's a great energy booster, has exceptional anti-inflammatory and anti-aging properties and strengthens your immune response. Finally, it's a great all-round body strengthener, giving your heart and circulation a boost and helping lower cholesterol.

If you're not managing to eat lots of green vegetables, then dehydrated barley grass is the convenient and nutritious answer. You can buy it from most health food stores. A 5g teaspoon is equivalent to 100g (4oz) of vegetables like raw spinach, kale, alfalfa sprouts or broccoli.

WHEATGRASS: POWER PACKED

The nutritional properties of wheatgrass are similar to barley grass, but since the actual wheatgrass is virtually indigestible, it needs to be juiced. You can buy a wheatgrass juicer or simply take the capsules, powders or tablets now widely available. Be warned that the taste of wheatgrass is rather pungent, almost medicinal. But the benefits are worth it. Research shows it's an excellent source of calcium, iron, magnesium, potassium, phosphorus and zinc. It's even been referred to as "the richest nutritional liquid known to man."

The health benefits of wheatgrass are many and varied: principally, it provides exceptional nourishment, restores the endocrine system, enhances immunity, assists digestion and promotes weight loss due to its high enzyme content and cleansing effect.

ALGAE: THE HIGHEST SOURCE

Algae was the first form of life on earth, and its power is immense. Algae provides virtually every essential vitamin, mineral, amino acid, enzyme and protein. It is probably the single highest source of nutrition in existence. And the real power of algae is that it's so easily digested. There are more than 30,000 species of algae, but for health purposes here are the most important types: wild blue-green algae, spirulina and chlorella.

WILD BLUE-GREEN ALGAE: THE MIRACLE SUPERFOOD

You can buy wild blue-green algae in your local health food store in a palatable liquid form, where it's mixed with apple juice. (It's also available as a powder, capsule or tablet.) It's perfect if you eat on the go, need to lose weight, feel tired all the time and so on. Even if you think you're healthy, I recommend it as a complete source of everything your body needs. Wild blue-green algae contains virtually every nutrient going: vitamins, minerals, amino acids, live enzymes and protein (60 percent protein, a more complete amino acid profile than beef or soybeans), and is the best food source of beta-carotene, B vitamins and chlorophyll. Algae can help you think better and improve your memory – tests have shown that children do better at school on it and it's also been linked with reversing the progression of Alzheimer's. It can strengthen your immunity, and help with viruses, colds and flu.

SPIRULINA: THE DIETER'S FRIEND

Spirulina is a cultivated or farmed micro-algae, with one of the richest protein contents of all natural foods. It contains 60 to 70 percent complete protein. Meat, on the other hand, consists of only about 25 percent complete protein. It's thought spirulina can help control blood sugar and cravings, so it is a key food for dieters and can be used to assist weight loss and as a general nutritional foundation. Mix 1 teaspoon in juice first thing in the morning for a refreshing wake-up call.

CHLORELLA: CHOLESTEROL CURBER

Chlorella is a freshwater algae. It is rich in a number of nutrients including: protein, vitamin B12, zinc, iron, chlorophyll and essential fatty acids. Studies have shown that chlorella can boost your immune system, reduce cholesterol and prevent hardening of the arteries, which can lead to heart attack and strokes. It is also available in supplement form of liquid and tablets or capsules.

BEE SUPERFOODS

THE BEE BY-PRODUCTS, ESSENTIALLY THOSE SUBSTANCES PRODUCED BY BEES, HAVE EXCEPTIONAL HEALING POWERS. THEY INCLUDE ROYAL JELLY, BEE POLLEN AND PROPOLIS.

ROYAL JELLY: THE REJUVENATOR

The queen bee lives almost exclusively on royal jelly; and lives about forty times longer than the rest of the bees. It's packed with a wonderful range of nutrients essential for boosting energy levels and combating stress.

Researchers have discovered royal jelly contains an antibiotic almost a quarter as active as penicillin, but without the side effects. They also found that royal jelly halts the growth of bacteria that cause pimples and stomach bugs. I prescribe royal jelly for patients wanting to conceive a baby. And boy has that been successful! It comes in liquid and capsules or royal jelly paste.

BEE POLLEN: THE CRÈME DE LA CRÈME

This is the Rolls-Royce of the bee by-products, and is one of the finest natural remedies around. This gold, powderlike substance is produced by flowering plants, gathered by bees and is a powerhouse of nutrients. It can be used to help fight allergies (particularly hay fever and sinusitis), chronic infections, prostate enlargement and nutritional deficiencies. It comes in pellets, capsules and powder form.

PROPOLIS: THE NATURAL ANTIBIOTIC

When you see bees busy at work in your garden, this is partly what they're collecting. It's a sticky material from the buds and bark of mostly poplar and fir trees. The bees use it to coat the outside of the hive for sterilization. Any predator entering their domain is stung to death, and embalmed with propolis to prevent decay. Propolis prevents bacteria from multiplying in an organism, so it can strengthen our immune system. Propolis also maintains and enhances the essential healthy bacteria. As a result, it is used to improve acne, skin ailments, cold sores and even arthritis because of its antifungal, antiseptic and anti-inflammatory qualities. You can get propolis in lozenges and tablets, or in liquid form.

SUPERFOOD HERBS
THESE ARE MY TOP 5 HERB SUPERFOODS.

1 ASTRAGALUS – ENERGY BODY TONIC

This is an all-round immune booster which improves digestion dramatically. It's a favorite with my patients, not just for its cold and flu fighting capabilities, but for its use in weight management and fighting fatigue.

2 NETTLE – BOWEL BUSTER

A cup of warm water followed by a cup of nettle tea first thing in the morning will get you going in the bowel department. Nettle also cleanses the liver and helps keep infections at bay. You can eat young nettle leaves in spring – they are rich in vitamins and minerals. Cook and use in the same way as spinach and use in salads – once cooked, the leaves no longer sting. When you're picking young nettles, remember to choose an area well away from roads and other pollutants. Alternatively drink 2 cups of nettle tea daily or take as a tincture. It's a superb pick-me-up in the middle of the day. For men with prostate problems, start drinking 2–3 cups daily.

3 ALOE VERA – DIGESTION RELIEVER

I use aloe for digestive disorders, bloating, gas and flatulence. Take approximately 1 tablespoon daily or follow directions on bottle. Mix with apple or other fruit juice for a more pleasant taste.

4 SIBERIAN GINSENG – STRESS COMBATTER

Ginseng is one of the oldest known herbal remedies, having been used as an energizing tonic for thousands of years. It's a rejuvenative herb that works by nourishing tired blood and helping the body adapt to stress. In clinical practice, I have found ginseng particularly beneficial to patients during or after illness and just after surgery for its restorative and anti-infection qualities. It is also excellent for preventing or alleviating jet lag. Drink as a tea, 1 cup daily, or take in capsule or tincture form.

5 ECHINACEA – LYMPH MOVER

Now available everywhere due to its soaring popularity in recent years, echinacea is a household name when it comes to warding off the common cold. The reason that I like it so much is because it moves the fluid inside the body called lymph. Lymph runs parallel to the bloodstream and carries toxins out of the body. Unless you exercise daily, lymph won't move enough. Echinacea can come to the rescue. Take in liquid or capsule form, for 2–3 week periods, then take a break.

SEA VEGETABLES

Seaweed has been eaten for thousands of years in the Orient. It's surprisingly tasty and I have even noticed that some supermarkets are now selling "crispy seaweeds" in their cooler sections.

Sea vegetables contain more minerals than any other food source. These sea veggies can contain up to ten times more calcium than milk and eight times as much iron as beef. There are three types, according to how much exposure to light they have received. Brown types of seaweed, now widely available in health food stores and Japanese and other Asian food outlets, include wakame (a constituent of miso soup), kombu and arame. Red seaweed, used as food, includes dulse (particularly linked with cholesterol reduction). Green seaweed includes nori (often used to wrap sushi). Seaweed is usually sold in dried form; all you need to do is rinse and soak it and it'll become soft again. It can be used to flavor all sorts of dishes. Try to incorporate seaweed into your diet a couple of times a week.

ARAME
Consists of brown stringy strands. Works well when cooked with root vegetables, such as squash, parsnips and yams. Just soak the arame for five minutes before you're ready to use.

DULSE
Red-purple color with smooth flat leaves. Unique spice-like nutty flavor, mild in taste and a great addition to salads as there's no need to cook it (be sure to wash it carefully).

NORI
Mostly from Japan, nori is probably best known for being wrapped around sushi. It varies in color and is sold in thin flat rectangular sheets. Add it to soups and rice dishes, or use it for making sushi. There's no need to soak it as it's ready to use.

WAKAME
It has a sweet flavor and you can actually use it in sandwiches instead of lettuce. Soak for five minutes.

HIJIKI
Black, firm and nutritionally rich but quite strong tasting. Soak for twenty minutes then rinse – you will only need a small amount as it swells up hugely.

KELP
Kelp is available in powder or tablet form if you don't like the idea of eating sea vegetables. It is also used as a seasoning.

KOMBU
Used for centuries as a flavor enhancer and food tenderizer, and makes food more digestible.

LEAFY SUPERFOODS

GREEN LEAFY VEGETABLES

Most people do not eat enough of these green leafies. Yet their nutritional values are immense. Recent studies have conclusively and definitively confirmed that populations with diets rich in green leafy vegetables run a far lower risk of heart disease and cancer.

EXCESS WEIGHT

For those who are overweight and want to shed those extra pounds, then eating dark green leafy vegetables will shed the weight. If you eat these veggies raw, that's even better. These green leafies are generally available throughout the year at your local supermarket or food store. Start to slowly introduce some of these power veggies into your daily routine.

GREEN LEAFY SUPERFOOD VEGGIES

- Arugula (rocket salad)
- Beet greens
- Sprouted broccoli seeds
- Chicory
- Collards
- Dandelion greens
- Endive and escarole
- Kale
- Kohlrabi

- Lettuce
- Mustard greens
- Parsley
- Spinach (If you have kidney stones, best to give this one a miss because of its high oxalic acid content.)
- Swiss chard
- Turnip greens
- Watercress

LIVE ENZYME-RICH FOOD

Fruits and vegetables are at their most healthful when they are eaten raw. The cooking process not only degrades some of the vital nutrients, vitamins and minerals, but heat destroys all of the life enhancing enzymes.

WHAT ARE ENZYMES?

Raw foods are packed with food enzymes. Enzymes are released as soon as you begin to chew. Enzymes are the essential catalysts for all the chemical reactions in your body — your digestion, your immunity and all other metabolic and regenerative processes. Without them, you would cease to function or exist. Think of them as your body's labor force involved in every biochemical and physiological function. You depend on them to walk, talk, breathe, digest food and function. For good health and a strong immune system, enzymes need to be plentiful and vital.

When enzyme activity is low, you are likely to feel tired and unwell. So clearly the level of enzyme content in your food is more than important — it's crucial.

ENZYME TYPES

1 METABOLIC

Metabolic enzymes occur naturally within your body and act as catalysts in all your bodily functions — eating, breathing, regulating metabolism and so on. You need these enzymes to stay slim and trim.

2 DIGESTIVE

Digestive enzymes are produced by our bodies. They are responsible for breaking down the food you eat, and metabolizing and absorbing all the nutrients. If we eat a diet of processed, junky food, we overtax our pancreas organ to produce more digestive enzymes. If the pancreas is too weak and unable to secrete enough enzyme molecules, it will rob other organs of critical, life-providing metabolic enzymes and will then change these into digestive enzymes. Once this happens, the simplest tasks such as thinking, talking, walking and even breathing will become difficult chores.

3 FOOD

Food enzymes help the digestive process. They must come from the foods we eat. All raw foods such as raw fruit, vegetables, raw nuts and especially live sprouted seeds are the food sources for food enzymes.

WHAT ARE SPROUTS?

Sprouts are essentially young green plants germinated from the seeds of almost any living vegetation which may include, but are not limited to, nuts, seeds, grains, beans, legumes, as well as various grasses such as barley grass or wheatgrass. Some of the most common sprouts are alfalfa, mung, radish, clover, aduki, garbanzo (chickpea), lentil, soybean, sunflower, millet, quinoa, buckwheat, fenugreek, wheat, barley, soy, corn, oats, green peas and lima, just to name a few. Essentially, any seed or bean equipped with the genetic fabric potential to reproduce the next generation of plant life is sproutable.

THE SUPERSTAR NUTRITIONAL STATUS OF SPROUTS

Sprouts are nutritional superstars. They contain a high concentrate of antioxidant nutrients that fight against the damage caused by free radicals. Free radicals are substances produced within our bodies that cause damage to cell tissue and accelerate the aging process. Sprouts are also packed with vitamins, minerals, protein, enzymes and fiber as well as two anti-aging constituents — RNA and DNA (nucleic acids) — that are only found in living cells.

BUT WHAT DOES SPROUTING MEAN?

Sprouting is the process of soaking, then germinating the seed, and finally eating the growing live sprouts. Each sprouting seed is packed with the nutritional energy needed to create a full-grown healthy plant.

Once the seed is soaked in water, a process necessary for sprouting, loads of enzymes are released. Upon germination, the seed rapidly absorbs water (from soaking) and swells to at least twice its original size.

Simultaneously, the nutrient content swells too. Finally, the germination process effectively predigests the seed, making digestion and assimilation of its nutrients easy so there is less likelihood of food allergies. The end result is a superfood with enormous levels of proteins, vitamins, minerals, trace minerals, fiber and enzymes in the most easily digestible form. By sprouting, you not only gain the benefits of the raw food, but also dramatically increase the nutrient content of these seeds and grains.

THE SCIENCE

- Sprouting significantly increases the activity of the enzymes. Dr. Gabriel Cousens (MD), in his book *Spiritual Nutrition*, points out that germinating and sprouting increase enzyme levels by 6–20 times, depending upon the specific plant.
- A study conducted at Yale University by Dr. Paul Barkholden found that B vitamins increased in sprouts by as much as 2,000 percent.
- Another study, at the University of Pennyslvania by Dr. Barry Mack, reported a general overall average vitamin increase of more than 500 percent when seeds are sprouted.
- Nucleic acids, the fundamental constituents required for all cell growth and regeneration, increased by 30 percent after sprouting seeds, as did mineral content.
- The protein content of almost any seed also increases by 15–30 percent when sprouted, according to Dr. Elson Hass (MD) in his book *Staying Healthy With Nutrition*.
- Professor of Nutritional Biochemistry at the University of Puget Sound, Dr. Jeffrey Bland showed that approximately 6 cups of sprouts could potentially supply the recommended daily nutritional intake for the average adult. Dr. Bland concluded that sprouts are a "more efficient, healthier form of protein than the conventional animal or even other types of vegetable proteins."

A KEY TO YOUR HEALTH

Eating sprouted foods regularly can result in dramatic improvements to digestion, immunity and your general health and well-being.

Not only will your digestion be healthy and your body more alkaline when you include sprouted foods in your diet on a regular basis, but you'll be better equipped to prevent and combat common colds and flu, illnesses, even dreaded diseases. Research has shown that sprouts help to keep the immune system strong. When the immune system is fortified, you are far less likely to be stricken – or to succumb to common or degenerative health ailments.

Consider the following study conducted by a team of researchers at the University of Texas Cancer Center. They found that the cancer cells were "99 percent inhibited" by the mix of live (sprouted) sprouts, mainly sprouted broccoli seeds. Statistically speaking, this would suggest that live sprouts may, in some cases, have the ability to inhibit cancer cells. Wow! At the clinic, I have had great success using sprouted broccoli seeds for patients who had been suffering from immune dysfunction. So if you are the type of person who is always catching the next cold or flu, then be sure to add lots of raw sprouts, especially sprouted broccoli seeds, to your daily regimen.

OUTSTANDING SPROUTS

You can literally sprout any seed, grain or legume for food in your own kitchen. The greatest health benefits come from sprouted millet and quinoa, as well as sprouted daikon and broccoli seeds.

The easiest sprouts to seed are:
► Aduki
► Alfalfa
► Clover
► Fenugreek (spicy)
► Green/red peas
► Lentils
► Mung beans
► Quinoa
► Radish
► Wheat

Also try:
► Chickpeas
► Sunflower seeds
► Broccoli seeds
► Millet

HOW TO SPROUT SEEDS AND BEANS

The easiest way to sprout seeds is to buy a sprouting kit and sprinkle water over the seeds. Try quinoa, broccoli seeds, clover, alfalfa seeds, mung beans, fenugreek and wheatberries, for example.

To do it yourself at home, all you need is a large jam jar, some seeds or beans, fresh water and a piece of cheesecloth or muslin.

► Rinse the seeds well. Place in the jar and cover with a half inch of cooled, boiled water. Cover with cheesecloth or net cloth secured with a rubber band and leave overnight in a warm, dark place.
► Rinse seeds next day with fresh water. Drain well or the seeds will rot. Return to the dark. Do this twice a day until seeds start to sprout. Tilt your jar to a 45-degree angle to allow the sprouts to grow up the jar.
► Then place them on a sunny windowsill for a few hours to get an energy boost. Eat or store in an airtight container in the fridge. Sprouts will keep in the fridge for 2–3 days.
► Refer to the sprouting chart on the next page and have fun with it. Take your time and enjoy the benefits.

SEEDS	SOAKING TIME (HOURS)	QUANTITY	YIELD
▸ Alfalfa	4–6	3tbsp	3 cups
▸ Amaranth	4–6	3tbsp	¾ cup
▸ Anise	4–6	3 tbsp	1 cup
▸ Barley	8–10	½ cup	1 cup
▸ Most beans	8–10	1 cup	3–4 cups
▸ Buckwheat	4–6	1 cup	2–3 cups
▸ Cabbage	4–6	1 tbsp	1½ cups
▸ Chia	4–6	1 tbsp	1½ cups
▸ Chickpeas	10–12	1 cup	3 cups
▸ Clover	4–6	1 tbsp	2½ cups
▸ Corn	8–10	1 cup	2 cups
▸ Fenugreek	4–6	4 tbsp	1 cup
▸ Flax	5–7	1 tbsp	1 cup
▸ Green peas	10–12	1 cup	2 cups
▸ Lentils	6–8	1 cup	3–4 cups
▸ Millet	6–8	1 cup	1½ cups
▸ Mung beans	8–10	1 cup	3–4 cups
▸ Mustard	4–6	1 tbsp	1 cup
▸ Most nuts	8–12	1 cup	1½ cups
▸ Oats	8–10	1 cup	2 cups
▸ Onion	4–6	1 tbs.	1 cup
▸ Quinoa	4–6	1 cup	2½ cups
▸ Radish	4–6	1 tbsp	1 cup
▸ Rice	8–10	1 cup	1½ cups
▸ Rye	8–10	1 cup	2½ cups
▸ Pumpkin seeds	6–8	1 cup	1½ cups
▸ Sesame seeds	4–6	1 cup	1½ cups
▸ Sunflower seeds	6–8	1 cup	1½ cups
▸ Soybeans	10–12	1 cup	2½ cups
▸ Watercress	4–6	1 tbsp	1½ cups
▸ Wheat	10–12	1 cup	2½ cups

THE CASE AGAINST COOKING

All raw foods and the sprouted seeds are the healthiest foods in existence. The raw foods are packed with life-enhancing enzymes, active vitamins, minerals, proteins and other micronutrients. Nutrients are degraded and all of the enzymes are destroyed when you cook, steam, bake, sauté, fry, roast, stew, boil or grill foods, or pasteurize or can them; virtually all the healthful properties disappear. Cooking does not improve the nutritional value of food. Heat makes up to 85 percent of nutrients unavailable and totally destroys the enzymes.

DESTRUCTION OF ENZYMES

When food is cooked, the enzymes are destroyed in full. Research has shown that when any food is heated above 118°F for approximately twenty minutes, there is complete and total devastation of all enzymes within that specific food.

LOSS OF PROTEIN

The process of cooking not only destroys enzymes, but protein too. Most protein is destroyed or converted to forms that are not easily digested. Studies sponsored by the United States Department of Agriculture concluded that "cooking at 400°F (the average temperature for cooking meats) caused a very marked decrease (4 to 30 fold) in the soluble protein of the steaks under analysis." Many of us think of meat as our main source of protein, but the fact is we are probably getting very little from our meat due to the high heat used in cooking.

LOST VITAMINS

As if the loss of enzymes and protein power isn't enough, vitamins are also damaged by the cooking process. Although not all vitamins are destroyed from high heat, studies have shown that vitamin activity is enormously curtailed. It is estimated that no less than 50 percent of B vitamins are lost through cooking. Some of the B vitamins are drastically reduced still further. For instance, the loss of thiamin (B1) can be as high as 96 percent if the food is boiled for a prolonged time. Similarly up to 72 percent of biotin can be lost, up to 97 percent of folic acid lost and up to 80 percent of vitamin C lost, all from cooking. In fact, according to one of the world's leading researchers on the topic, Dr. Viktoras Kulvinskas, in his *Survival Report into the 21st Century*, there is an average overall "nutrient destruction of approximately 85 percent from cooking." In other words, when food is cooked we are often getting less than 15 percent of the nutritive value of the food, a lesser percentage of protein and zero percent of the enzymes.

OTHER HOT ISSUES

Eating very hot food isn't good news for your bodily functions either. It can cause other enzymatic problems. For example, research has shown that stomach upsets are likely if you drink beverages that are simply too hot. Too hot food (in temperature) also poses risk of gum problems, mouth ulcers and tongue and throat cancers.

One of the most alarming studies by medical researchers found that a diet full of cooked foods may cause the reduction of brain tissue and the swelling of the key organs. Cooked food also overworks the endocrine glands. The endocrine system, along with the nervous system, regulates appetite. If your endocrine glands know you've had enough calories, but nutrients and enzymes are missing from the foods, then your body will keep demanding more food just to keep its strength up. The result may be weight problems, exhaustion and poor health.

The overeating of cooked food also compromises the overall immune system. Cooked foods have been shown to actually adversely alter blood structure. In my own live cell analysis of patients' blood work, I have found that the people who only eat cooked foods have blood cells that appear to be in a constant state of alert (as if they were fighting a constant infection). In effect, the white blood cells become overworked, a condition known as "leukocytosis." This is incredibly weakening to the immune system.

Immunity may no longer be able to perform when a real infection sets in. It's like constantly revving your car engine; eventually it gets flooded and won't start at all. In this sense, cooked foods flood your blood system, the immune system and the organs.

BALANCING ACT

The good news here, however, is that the presenting researcher at the International Congress of Microbiology, Dr. Paul Kouchakoff (MD), emphatically pointed out that eating raw foods, or even just foods heated below 190°F, could prevent any rise in white blood cells. Perhaps most significantly, though, was that Dr. Kouchakoff found that eating an approximate 50–50 ratio (50 percent raw foods to 50 percent cooked foods) could also prevent leukocytosis. You don't need to go cold turkey on cooking or eating hot food entirely. You can still eat cooked foods, but you just need to balance them with some raw.

Although I want you to know the benefits of increasing your intake of raw fruits, vegetables and sprouts, I am not advocating that you eat all raw all the time. Instead I am saying that you should (a) eat more raw; and (b) whenever you eat a cooked food, balance it with some raw foods. The combination of cooked with raw foods is the best.

GETTING IN THE RAW

So when you fancy something cooked, whenever possible it is better to warm the foods rather than vigorously cook them. For instance, you obviously need to do some cooking if you want to have soup. But you can still manage to get in the raw. Once the soup is hot and ready to serve, you can add various fresh raw vegetables to the soup just moments before it hits the table. In this way, you can enjoy warm soup in the winter knowing you're still getting a substantial ration of raw (completely uncooked) vegetables contained within the soup.

WARMING FOODS

A useful tip to help you cut down on cooking is to include more warming foods which warm the body, whether served raw, cold or warm. For example: cinnamon, garlic, quinoa sprouts or ginger are "warming herbs." These foods also serve an important function in our bodies, helping to circulate the blood and comfort the organs.

WARMING HERBS/ SEASONING
Basil, bay leaves, caraway, cardamom, chives, cinnamon, cloves, coriander, cumin, dill, fennel, fenugreek, garlic, ginger, lemongrass, mustard, nutmeg, oregano, pepper, spearmint

WARMING SPROUTS
Fenugreek sprouts, radish sprouts

THE BOTTOM LINE
Most of us simply do not eat enough raw foods. You don't have to cut out all cooked food altogether. You just need to include more raw foods in your daily diet. When you do cook, go for warm rather than hot. Raw food and sprouts provide us with a broader range of active nutrients and enzymes than any other way of eating. Don't deprive yourself of all their life-giving and health-boosting properties. My message is simple: Eat less of the cooked, and more of the raw.

CONCLUSION

You now know just how true it is that "You Are What You Eat." But too often, something deep within each of us prevents us from eating the right foods, even though we know we need to if we want to look and feel great. I believe the answer to this lies within the emotional, psychological and physical constraints we create for ourselves when it comes to new ideas and a new lifestyle. Most, after all, are afraid of change. Trust me; I was just like that at one time too.

I hope that within these pages I have gone some way to opening you up to these changes, however small at first. I would like to share with you my advice for how to become more accepting of new ideas, new foods, a new lifestyle, and the owner of an amazing healthy body too!

Once you understand the powerful nature of energy, you will appreciate the impact of my advice. All weight problems, eating disorders, lethargy, disease and illness have their roots, in some form, in the disturbance of energy. Positive energy flow and good foods will keep you strong and healthy. Negative energy flow and poor food choices will make you tired and sick.

The bottom line here is that in order to achieve great health, youthful spirit and a fantastic body, I want you to be happy, positive and fun-loving. I'd like to leave you, therefore, with two key simple and easy points of advice to infuse positivity into your cells:

FIRST: BE PROACTIVE, NOT REACTIVE

We can choose to simply react to our environment or we can make the conscious decision to act with direction, purpose and in search of fulfillment. You become the creator of situations, instead of the reactor. You become the cause, instead of the effect.

You become happy and healthy.

Next time you feel like life is challenging you and poses a threat to your natural sense of balance, try working through the following steps:

- Recognize that a difficult situation has arisen.
- Acknowledge that the purpose of this challenge is to help, teach and assist you.
- See the difficulty not as a victim's sour grapes, but as a gift to improve your life.
- Identify your reaction or potential reaction. What are you feeling? Acknowledge those feelings and accept them as being okay.
- Take a nice long inhalation of breath. While doing so, imagine a beautiful golden white light entering your body and enveloping you. As you exhale, visualize all of the negative feelings leaving you.
- On your next inhalation, allow a sense of calm to enter your body. As you exhale, tell yourself to release all negative reactive behavior and feelings.
- Now take action. Deal with your difficult situation in a proactive way. Act with clarity, certainty and calm.

SECOND: LOVE UNCONDITIONALLY

Finally, this is my deepest secret to achieving great health and a fantastic life. Yes, you are what you eat. But just as integral is that you are what you love. After many years of biochemical study, molecular research, clinical practice and living life, I have discovered that the most powerful energetic influence for good health is the energy force of love.

Love is the strongest driving force for the body's energetic balance, healing process, disease prevention, cellular rejuvenation, organ vitality, blood cleansing, molecular revitalization and virbrational freedom. So just remember to love yourself, your body and the people in your life, especially the stranger a yonder and a hug for your loved ones too.

Wishing you love and light always, see you next time,

Gillian

DR. GILLIAN MCKEITH

Dr. Gillian McKeith (Ph.D.) is a global phenomenon. Hailed the "World's Most Acclaimed Nutritionist" by the *Daily Mail* (London), Dr. McKeith is an internationally renowned clinical nutritionist and the director of the McKeith Research Centre in London.

She works wonders for patients who come to consult with her from all regions of the world and from all walks of life, including Hollywood stars, professional athletes, and members of the royal family. Gillian is the presenter of *You Are What You Eat*, the smash hit national prime-time TV series in the United Kingdom that is now being broadcast in dozens of countries throughout the world. She is also the author of the number-one bestselling book *You Are What You Eat*, which has sold more than two million copies in the UK alone. The book is now being translated into other languages around the globe. She is also author of *Living Food For Health* (Piatkus/Basic), and *Miracle Superfood: Wild Blue-Green Algae* (McGraw Hill).

Dr. Gillian graduated from the University of Edinburgh and received her master's degree from the University of Pennsylvania in Philadelphia. After a severe bout of personal ill health and recovery through nutritional medicine, she embarked upon a new path and changed her life. She then spent several years re-training for a master's and doctorate (Ph.D.) in holistic nutrition from the American Holistic College of Nutrition (U.S.). She holds certificates from the London School of Acupuncture and the Kailish Centre of Oriental Medicine. She is currently studying with the Australasian College Of Health Sciences, U.S.A. She is a postgraduate member of the Centre For Nutrition Education in England and is a member of several health organizations in the UK and U.S. Raised in Scotland, Gillian now travels extensively, giving lectures and seminars to packed audiences.

Her lifelong mission is to share her information and improve people's lives everywhere.

www.drgillianmckeith.com

INDEX

ACKNOWLEDGMENTS

Heartfelt gratitude to Howard White, Esq., for placing and helping me on the path for this journey, for sharing your clairvoyance, for your words and immense impact on my life. I am forever grateful to Marian Moore for sharing with me her gift of healing. A special thank you to Badiene who introduced me to sprouts (not Brussels) and so much more. In memory of Auntie Rita who impressed upon me the importance of helping others to help themselves. I am forever grateful to Doug and Eloise for their cataclysmic wisdom and for always being there for me.

Thanks to:
Alan Martin for doing so much behind the scenes with our TV participants. Theresa Cheung and Sarah Wilson for your cutting edge research, and Paula Bartimeus too. Nicola Ibison for seeing my vision and giving it your all. Julia, Helen, Jo and everyone at NCI Management. Luigi Bonomi at Sheil Land for your out of this world skills. Smith & Gilmour for fantastic book design, Gillian Haslam for editing and Ken Townson for the back cover photo. And to Kate Adams and all at Penguin for their tremendous support.

Special thanks to everyone at Celador Productions Ltd, including: Anna Richardson for your contribution in development of the series *You Are What You Eat* and for having the vision to know that I could do it; Paul Smith and Danielle Lux for this wonderful opportunity to share health information with the nation; Damon Pattison for your guidance, support and great sense of humor; Claire Masters for pulling it all together and making it happen; Linda Brusasco, Gavin Searle and Diane Elkins for your creative genius and direction; Mary Paraskakis, Lucy Taylor, Helen Wood, Claire Mills, Badannie Grant, Jessica Owen, Rosie Gratton and Danielle Thornton for all your hard work; Justine Pattison and Angie Platt for delicious food preparation of both good foods and bad foods; Perry Harrison, Stuart Burroughs and Rob Entwhistle for great camera and sound. Many thanks to everyone else involved in this book and TV program preparation.

Appreciation to Chaim Solomon for your no-nonsense advice and spiritual teachings to keep me on track.

Love and thanks to Mum and Dad for their support too.